Y. Kusaka, K.G. Hering, J.E. Parker (Eds.)

International Classification of HRCT for Occupational and Environmental Respiratory Diseases

Y. Kusaka, K.G. Hering, J.E. Parker (Eds.)

International Classification of HRCT for Occupational and Environmental Respiratory Diseases

With 94 Figures, including 27 in Color

Springer

Yukinori Kusaka, M.D., Ph.D.
Industrial Health Consultant
Professor and Chairman
Department of Environmental Health, School of Medicine
Fukui Medical University
23-3 Shimoaizuki, Matsuoka-cho, Fukui 910-1193, Japan

Kurt G. Hering, M.D.
Chief
Department of Diagnostic Radiology, Radiooncology and Nuclear Medicine
Radiologische Klinik, Knappschaftskrankenhaus, Dortmund
Wieckesweg 27, 44309 Dortmund, Germany

John E. Parker, M.D.
Professor
Pulmonary and Critical Care Medicine
Robert C. Byrd Health Sciences Center, West Virginia University
HSC 475A-9166, Morgantown, West Virginia 26506-9166, U.S.A.

Cover Illustration: From Georgius Agricola (1556) *De Re Metallica*, Herbert Clark Hoover and Lou Henry Hoover, translators (1950) Dover Publications, Inc., New York, with permission

This book was financially supported by the Japan Society for the Promotion of Science (Grant-in-Aid for Publication of Scientific Research Result: Grant No. 165303).

Additional material to this book can be downloaded from http://extras.springer.com.

ISBN 4-431-23924-3 Springer-Verlag Tokyo Berlin Heidelberg New York

Library of Congress Control Number: 2004117722

Printed on acid-free paper

Springer-Verlag is a part of Springer Science+Business Media
springeronline.com

Typesetting: Camera-ready by the editors and authors
Printing and binding: Shinano Inc., Japan

Foreword

Environmental and occupational exposure to mineral dusts (i.e., pneumoconiosis) has long been known to be an important cause of lung disease. Since the latter half of the twentieth century, the number of pneumoconiosis cases recognized by physicians has increased significantly, related to both an increased likelihood of exposure to toxic materials in industry and more detailed surveillance of workers.

Our ability to diagnose and subsequently avoid, control, and regulate these harmful exposures has been based on understanding their relationship to clinical symptoms and pathologic lung abnormalities. Fundamental to this understanding has been the widely used system for classification of chest radiographic abnormalities in pneumoconiosis introduced by the International Labour Office (ILO). Based on this system, the type and degree of lung abnormality could be readily assessed in a population of exposed subjects, and correlations made with exposure severity or duration, morbidity, and mortality. However, the limitations of the ILO system have long been recognized. Chest radiographs are insensitive to the diagnosis of early abnormalities produced by pneumoconioses, and they lack specificity as well; a number of findings considered abnormal on chest radiographs using ILO criteria are in fact nonspecific and may not be related to pneumoconiosis at all.

The development of high-resolution computed tomography (HRCT) over the last 20 years has revolutionized the diagnosis of all types of lung disease, including pneumoconiosis. The anatomic detail provided by HRCT, in combination with detailed correlations of HRCT lung abnormalities and histologic findings, has provided a powerful tool for assessment of these diseases. However, a comprehensive system for the classification and quantification of the lung abnormalities typically seen in patients with pneumoconiosis has been lacking. Without question, a HRCT system for the classification and quantification of pneumoconiosis, similar to the ILO system, would be valuable in our attempts to accurately diagnose and effectively prevent these diseases.

This monograph provides just such a system. Based on a fundamental understanding of HRCT, both its technical aspects and anatomic correlations, the authors have provided a detailed and comprehensive description of significant HRCT findings and methods for appropriately recording them. They have considered all aspects of the HRCT diagnosis of pneumoconiosis, including the technical aspects of CT, radiation exposure and risks associated with HRCT, the use of appropriate terminology in the description of abnormalities, coding systems (including a review of the ILO system), and pathologic correlations, and they also provide reference standards for diagnosis. This work is based on the conclusions of an international meeting of experts in lung imaging and pneumoconiosis diagnosis held in Nikko, Japan, and subsequently refined by investigators from countries around the world; it thus represents the contributions of a number of experts in this field. It is a major step in our ability to assess pneumoconiosis.

W. Richard Webb, M.D.
Professor of Radiology
Chief, Thoracic Imaging
University of California, San Francisco
January 2005

Preface

Modern medical textbooks are rarely single-author efforts; rather, they are more often the products of multi-author scientific cooperation. This volume is no exception to that trend, and the work is indeed an example of the international collaboration required to produce a text with global relevance. Brought together here are unique contributions from many nations on several continents, and the true catalyst has been the steady encouragement of Japanese colleagues.

This work represents an international journey, an odyssey with historical parallels that are interesting to reflect upon. Ancient Japan was known for its gold trade. Refined gold was transported through China to the Netherlands and then to the rest of Europe. In fact, Japan was called Jipang, meaning literally, Golden Hope Island. This book is the golden fruit of the hope and work of many medical scientists.

Nikko, the famous Japanese city, originally located near a gold mine opened in the early fifteenth century, was the auspicious location and memorable site where international experts from Germany, Finland, the United States, and Japan agreed on a principal coding system, along with reference films and imaging parameters. This work, referred to as the Nikko Agreement, has been the cornerstone for the International Classification of High-Resolution Computed Tomography for Occupational and Environmental Respiratory Diseases.

Subsequently, British, French, and Belgian colleagues worked together in Dortmund, Germany, to further refine the classification system. Ultimately, colleagues from seven countries collaborated in the development of this project.

In many cultures, traditional phrases have suggested that too many cooks can spoil the soup, or make it too salty. However, also recognizing seven as a lucky number in many societies, colleagues from seven countries have managed to create a wonderful product from this collaboration and have indeed produced quite a tasty soup. The international flavor of the project is further exemplified by reading trials of candidate HRCT films with as many as 25 colleagues from the seven countries. In addition, reviews, comments, and suggestions for the further refinement of the classification system have also come from Sweden, Norway, Denmark, Switzerland, the Czech Republic, Brazil, Malaysia, India, Vietnam, Thailand, Korea, and China.

The editors would like to acknowledge the hard work and contributions of many colleagues around the globe. We dedicate this book, and also wish to express our gratitude to, three life-long collaborators closer to our respective homes and dear to our hearts, our wives: Mrs. Johanna Hering, Mrs. Junko Kusaka, and

Mrs. Christine Parker. Without their support this project would not have become a reality, and the soup would have indeed been far too salty.

Yukinori Kusaka
Kurt G. Hering
John E. Parker

Acknowledgement

We would like to thank the following experts for developing this classification:

Drs. Thomas Kraus, Siegfied Tuengerthal, Tapio Vehmas, Leena Kivisaari, Hiroaki Arakawa, Masanori Akira, Hisao Shida, Harumi Itoh, Yutaka Hosoda, Narufumi Suganuma, Yasuo Nakajima, Yomei Hiraga, Michael Crane, Marc Letourneux, and Pierre A. Gevenois

We thank Mr. Takashi Ogura, Canon Inc. for preparing images of the reference CT films.

We also thank the following experts for participating the validity study on the reference CT films:

Drs. Tarja Routsalainen, Daniel A. Henry, Ralph T. Shipley, Lee Sider, David A. Lynch, Sian Phillips, Huw Roach, Jacques Ameille, Jean-Pierre Bertrand, Pietro Scillia, and P. De Vuyst.

Yukinori Kusaka
Kurt G. Hering
John E. Parker

Contents

Contributors

Name of Author (Chapter)

Masanori Akira, Dr. (Chapter 8)
Chief
Department of Radiology, National Kinki Central Hospital
1180 Nagasone-cho, Sakai
Osaka 591-8025, Japan
Tel: +81-722-52-3021
Fax: +81-722-51-1372

Hiroaki Arakawa, Dr. (Chapters 1, 9)
Assistant Professor
Department of Radiology, Dokkyo University School of Medicine
880 Oaza-Kitakobayashi, Mibu-cho, Shimotsuga-gun
Tochigi 321-0207, Japan
Tel: +81-282-87-2171
Fax: +81-282-86-4940
E-mail: arakawa@dokkyomed.ac.jp

Michael D. Crane, Dr. (Chapter 7)
Consultant Radiologist
Radiology Department, Llandough Hospital
Penlan Road, Near Penarth, Glamorgan CF64 2XX
Wales, U.K.
Tel: +44-29-20-711711
Fax: +44-29-20-708973
E-mail: M.D.Crane@btinternet.com

Pierre A. Gevenois, Dr. (Chapter 7)
Professor
Department of Radiology, Hospital Erasme-Universite Libre de Bruxelles
Route de Leinnik 808 1070
Bruxelles, Belgium
Tel: +32-2-555-3220
Fax: +32-2-555-4388
E-mail: pier.alan.gevenois@ulb.ac.be

Kurt G. Hering, Dr. (Introduction, Chapter 2, CD-ROM)
Chief
Department of Diagnostic Radiology, Radiooncology and Nuclear Medicine
Radiologische Klinik, Knappschaftskrankenhaus, Dortmund
Wieckesweg 27
44309 Dortmund, Germany
Tel: +49-231-922-0/1600
Fax: +49-231-201721
E-mail: k.g.hering@t-online.de

Koichi Honma, Dr. (Chapter 9)
Associate Professor
Department of Pathology, Dokkyo University School of Medicine
880 Oaza-Kitakobayashi, Mibu-cho, Shimotsuga-gun
Tochigi 321-0207, Japan
Tel: +81-282-86-1111
Fax: +81-282-86-5678
E-mail: homma@dokkyomed.ac.jp

Yutaka Hosoda, Dr. (Chapters 6, 9)
Consultant
Radiation Effects Research Foundation
1-41-4 Higashinakano, Nakano-ku
Tokyo 164-0003, Japan
Tel: +81-3-3361-3104
Fax: +81-3-3361-3104
E-mail: yhosoda@mvj.biglobe.ne.jp

Harumi Itoh, Dr. (CD-ROM)
Professor and Chairman
Department of Radiology, School of Medicine, Fukui Medical University
23-3 Shimoaizuki, Matsuoka-sho
Fukui 910-1193, Japan
Tel: +81-776-61-8368
Fax: +81-776-61-8137
E-mail: hitoh@fmsrsa.fukui-med.ac.jp

Juhani Karppinen, Dr. (Chapter 4)
Radiation and Nuclear Safety Authority
P.O. Box14, FIN 00881
Helsinki, Finland
E-mail: juhani.karppinen@stuk.fi

Leena Kivisaari, Dr. (Chapter 3)
Professor
Department of Radiology, Helsinki University Central Hopital
Haartmaninkatu 4, P.O. Box 380, FIN-00029
Helsinki, Finland
E-mail: Leena.Kivisaari@huch.fi

Thomas Kraus, Dr. (Chapter 2)
Institute and Outpatient Clinic for Occupational Medicine
University Hospital Aachen
Pauwelsstr. 30, D-52074
Aachen, Germany
Tel: +49-241 80 88880
Fax: +49-241 80 82587
E-mail: Thomas.Kraus@post.rwth-aachcn.dc

Yukinori Kusaka, Dr. (Introduction, Chapter 5)
Industrial Health Consultant
Professor and Chairman
Department of Environmental Health, School of Medicine
Fukui Medical University
23-3 Shimoaizuki, Matsuoka-cho
Fukui 910-1193, Japan
Tel: +81-776-61-8338
Fax: +81-776-61-8107
E-mail: yukik@fmsrsa.fukui-med.ac.jp

Marc Letourneux, Dr. (Chapter 7)
Professor
Service de medicine du travail et pathologie professionnelle
Niveau 1-CHU Cote deu Nacre
14033 Caen Cedex, France
Tel: +33-2-31-06-45-89
Fax: +33-2-31-06-49-14
E-mail: letourneux-m@chu-caen.fr

Kanae Nishizawa, Dr. (Chapter 4)
Medical Exposure Assessment Section
Department of Medical Physics, National Institute of Radiological Sciences
4-9-1 Anagawa, Inage-ku
Chiba 263-8555, Japan
Tel: +81-43-206-3064
Fax: +81-43-284-0918
E-mail: nisizawa@nirs.go.jp

John E. Parker, Dr. (Introduction)
Professor
Pulmonary and Critical Care Medicine
Robert C. Byrd Health Sciences Center, West Virginia University
HSC 475A-9166, Morgantown
West Virginia 26506-9166, U.S.A.
Tel: +1-304-293-4661
Fax: +1-304-293-3724
E-mail: parker@labyrinth.net/jparker@hsc.wvu.edu

Hisao Shida, Dr. (Chapter 9)
Senior Lecturer
Rosai Hospital for Silicosis, Labor Welfare Corporation
632 Takatoku, Fujiwara-machi, Shioya-gun
Tochigi 321-2523, Japan
Tel: +81-288-76-1515
Fax: +81-288-76-1611
E-mail: shida@keihai.gr.jp

Narufumi Suganuma, Dr. (Chapter 5)
Lecturer
Department of Environmental Health, School of Medicine
Fukui Medical University
23-3 Shimoaizuki, Matsuoka-cho
Fukui 910-1193, Japan
Tel: +81-776-61-8338
Fax: +81-776-61-8107
E-mail: suganuma@fmsrsa.fukui-med.ac.jp

Tapio Vehmas, Dr. (Chapters 3, 4)
Senior Lecturer
Radiology Unit, Finnish Institute of Occupational Health
Topeliuksenkatu 41aA, FIN-00250
Helsinki, Finland
Tel: +358-9-4747-481
Fax: +358-9-2412-414
E-mail: tapio.vehmas@occuphealth.fi

Shinji Yoshinaga, Dr. (Chapter 4)
Environmental Radiation Protection Research Group
Research Center for Radiation Safety
National Institute of Radiological Sciences
4-9-1 Anagawa, Inage-ku
Chiba 263-8555, Japan
Tel: +81-43-206-3108
Fax: +81-43-251-6089
E-mail: yosinaga@nirs.go.jp

Introduction

Yukinori Kusaka[1], Kurt G. Hering[2], and John E. Parker[3]

[1] Department of Environmental Health, School of Medicine, Fukui Medical University, 23-3 Shimoaizuki, Matsuoka-cho, Fukui 910-1193, Japan

[2] Department of Diagnostic Radiology, Radiooncology and Nuclear Medicine, Radiologische Klinik, Knappschaftskrankenhaus, Dortmund, Wieckesweg 27, 44309 Dortmund, Germany

[3] Pulmonary and Critical Care Medicine, Robert C. Byrd Health Sciences Center, West Virginia University, HSC 475A-9166, Morgantown, West Virginia 26506-9166, U.S.A.

Mineral dust-related lung diseases, the pneumoconiosis, have been recognized for centuries, and these diseases are especially common since global industrialization. Recently, not only occupational, but also environmental exposures to asbestos have been recognized throughout the world. Accordingly, industrialized nations will face the highest numbers of asbestos-related pulmonary diseases including malignant mesothelioma, over next few decades. Although the International Labour Office Classification System for the Pneumoconioses is widely used, it is designed for conventional analogue chest radiographs.

New modalities in the radiological sciences continue to be developed. Computed Tomography (CT) including High-Resolution CT has revolutionized the diagnostic universe of chest diseases, especially for lung cancer and diffuse lung disease. Clinical radiology has used the advantages of CT and continues to explore the potential of CT to provide exquisite imaging details of the thorax. The same advantages of CT can be used to study the pneumoconioses, also disorders representing forms of diffuse interstitial lung disease. CT is thus a potential tool for both clinical and epidemiological evaluation of dust diseases. Recently, trials for lung cancer screening with CT in a variety of populations have been implemented.

The primary disadvantage of chest CT over analogue radiographs is higher radiation exposure. Despite this disadvantage, surveillance and screening with CT may compete favorably as a tool with conventional radiography, especially if a standardized approach to classification using low dose CT, analogous to the ILO System for traditional radiographs, is widely available. The International Classification of High-Resolution Computed Tomography for Occupational and Environmental Respiratory Diseases has been developed and now introduced by physicians active in the recognition and prevention of dust diseases.

The International Classification of High-Resolution Computed Tomography for Occupational and Environmental Respiratory Diseases can assist in diagnostic evaluations of dust-exposed individuals. The Classification also provides a tool for quantitative and analytical measurement of disease, and can contribute to medical epidemiology.

The International Classification of High-Resolution Computed Tomography for Occupational and Environmental Respiratory Diseases is a powerful and reliable tool for international clinicians and scientists who study pulmonary fibrosis and malignancy.

Part I

Classification System

Chapter 1 A Glossary of HRCT Terms

Hiroaki Arakawa

Department of Radiology, Dokkyo University School of Medicine, 880, Shimo-tuga-gun, Tochigi 321-0207, Japan

In this chapter we provide a quick reference for HRCT terms used in this coding system. The terms are used in a similar fashion as for non-occupational diseases. However, due to the variability of common usage of HRCT terminology, we attempt to clarify the meaning of the terms used in this coding system. The readers can use the following descriptive terms for occupational lung diseases as well for non-occupational lung diseases.

Air trapping

Abnormal gas retention in the lung specifically diagnosed by use of post-expiratory CT (1). It should not be used based on the observation of inspiratory CT scan only. The presence of air trapping is suggested by no or little increases of lung attenuation *and* cross-sectional area change before and after exhalation. Therefore, for the accurate diagnosis of air trapping, both inspiratory and expiratory images at the same or similar anatomical levels are required.

Alveolar pattern

Alveolar pattern is one of the radiographic descriptions of abnormal increase in lung attenuation seen with CT. Pathologically, airspace and most peripheral air conduction portions are filled with inflammatory exudate or tumor cells. On CT, alveolar pattern is seen as slightly increased lung attenuation area (ground-glass opacity) or homogeneously increased dense opacity with or without airbronchogram (consolidation). However, CT description of alveolar pattern is used confidently only when abnormally increased lung attenuation is accompanied with air bronchogram.

Bronchial wall thickening (BR)

Bronchial wall thickening is subjectively diagnosed. Comparison of the bronchial wall diameter with that of the adjacent pulmonary artery may be helpful. Because bronchial wall thickening and bronchiectasis are often multifocal rather than diffuse, comparison of the bronchial wall of concern with those of other lung areas can also be helpful.

Bronchovascular bundle (structure)

Pathologically, the brochovascular bundle is a strong connective sheath around bronchi and central pulmonary vessels that begins at the pulmonary hilum and spreads peripherally. On CT, soft tissue density surrounding bronchi and central vessels is called the bronchovascular bundle.

Bronchiectasis/bronchiolectasis (BE)

Bronchiectasis and bronchiolectasis are localized or diffuse dilatation of bronchi or bronchioles, respectively. On CT, bronchiectasis and bronchiolectasis are diagnosed on the combination of the following (2): 1) inner diameter of bronchi is larger than that of the accompanying pulmonary artery, 2) loss of normal tapering of bronchial lumen, 3) a bronchiole visible within 1cm of the pleura and 4) bronchial wall thickening. Because bronchial diameters often exceed that of the accompanying pulmonary artery even in normals, the diagnosis should not be made only on the size criteria (3).

Bulla (BU)

Bullae are well-demarcated air-filled spaces with a thin wall larger than 1cm. They are a specific form of a lung cyst. Bullae are usually associated with the presence of emphysema but can be present in the absence of emphysema.

Coalescence

Coalescence is the term used for a group of pneumoconiotic nodules gathering in a specific area of lung and forming a nearly single mass, but each nodule is still individually identifiable.

Centrilobular

Centrilobular is the adjective meaning the center of each secondary lobule. The centrilobular area includes pulmonary arteries and bronchioles as well as supporting connective tissue of bronchovascular interstitium. On CT, abnormalities in centrilobular location may be identified as a dot, nodule or binary branching structure depending on the pathologic processes creating the abnormality. One can recognize the abnormality as located centrilobular when one of the followings are identified (4): 1) the opacity is a few millimeters away from the pleura and/or septal lines, 2) the opacity is contiguous with peripheral pulmonary artery or bronchiole, 3) opacities are separated about 1cm with each other.

Comet tail appearance

See Rounded atelectasis.

Cyst

Cyst is a nonspecific word that describes well-circumscribed air-/fluid-filled space larger than 1cm. The wall is smooth and well-defined and is usually thin, although thick wall such as in honeycomb cyst is included.

Dependent opacity (DO)

Dependent opacity on CT, is the increased lung attenuation in the dependent portion of each lower lung and is seen in normal individuals even without an underlying pathologic process. This phenomenon is considered to be associated with the loss of air in alveoli due to gravity and should not be mistaken as ground-glass opacity. Because early interstitial abnormality can occur in the dorsal portion of lower lobes in asbestosis, prone position is preferred to avoid difficulty in discriminating the pathologic process and gravity dependent opacity in this coding system.

Diffuse pleural thickening

Diffuse pleural thickening is the condition where both parietal and visceral pleurae are affected by fibrous thickening. Pleural thickening is said to be diffuse only when there is also adjacent pulmonary parenchymal fibrosis recognizable on CT.

In this coding system, diffuse pleural thickening is called visceral type pleural thickening.

Eggshell calcification (ES)

Eggshell calcification is seen in silicosis and mixed dust pneumoconiosis, the enlargement of hilar and/or mediastinal lymph nodes is common. Calcification in lymph nodes often occurs and is preferentially in periphery, giving the appearance of eggshell. This type of calcification may also be seen in other diseases such as sarcoidosis, tuberculosis, and after radiation treatment for mediastinal lymphoma.

Emphysema (EM)

Emphysema is abnormal permanent enlargement of the airspaces distal to the terminal bronchioles, accompanied by destruction of their walls and without obvious fibrosis (5). On CT, emphysema is identified as cystic airspace usually without visible walls.

Grade

In this coding system, we **grade** the severity of each abnormality in its extent and consistency. Grade is scored with a four-point scale with the most severe grade as 3 and absence of abnormality as grade zero. Each grade is explained simply in the text and is accompanied by images of reference CT films.

Ground-glass opacity

Ground glass opacity is a hazy increase of lung attenuation that does not obscure underlying vessels. This is a non-specific descriptor of HRCT finding and both interstitial and alveolar abnormalities can cause this appearance.

Honeycombing

Honeycombing in the lung parenchyma is characterized by clustering of thick-walled cystic spaces. The thick walls are typically covered with bronchiolar epithelium (6). It is usually bilateral and identified in the subpleural areas of lower lungs. It is regarded as the result of end-stage pulmonary fibrosis of any etiology.

Inhomogeneous attenuation

Inhomogeneous attenuation is the visual impression of lung attenuation with intervening areas of higher and lower attentuations. Mosaic perfusion and ground-glass attenuation both can cause such appearances. Before deciding mosaic perfusion or ground-glass attenuation, one can just describe the presence of inhomogeneous lung attenuation in this coding system.

Intralobular opacity

See Irregular opacity.

Interlobular septal line

See Irregular opacity.

Irregular opacity

Irregular opacity comprises two distinct opacities; that is, interlobular opacity and intralobular opacity. Interlobular opacity is synonymous with thickening of interlobular septal line or Kerley's line. Interlobular opacity is often irregularly thickened in pneumoconiosis due to fibrosis or shows nodular appearance due to existing pneumoconiotic nodules. The opacity is linear and polygonal with a diameter 1-2cm apart.

Intralobular opacity is an irregular or reticular opacity seen within a secondary lobule. It is finer than interlobular opacity and can be seen anywhere within secondary lobule. In asbestosis, it represents fibrosis and collapse of peribronchiolar interstitium and surrounding alveoli (7). Although centrilobular binary structure or dot in p-type silicosis can simulate intralobular opacity, they are not included in irregular opacity and should be recorded as rounded opacity due to their original nature to form nodules.

Large opacity

A large opacity is a nodular or mass-like opacity more than 1 cm in largest diameter. It is subcategorized depending on the summation of their size. Pneumoconiotic opacity as well as nodules or masses of other etiology are included as a large opacity. However, rounded atelectasis is excluded and should not be described as large opacity in this coding system.

Macule

Macule is an accumulation of dust-laden macrophages at the centrilobular interstitium forming a colored nodule on cutting. On CT, macule is not typically visible because of lack of fibrosis.

Lung distortion (DI)

Lung distortion means an irreversible displacement of normal pulmonary structures due to lung fibrosis. On CT, one can recognize the abnormality when pulmonary vessels, inter-lobar fissures, bronchi or mediastinal structures are displaced irregularly in or near the area with reticular and ground-glass opacities.

Mosaic perfusion (MP)

Mosaic perfusion, is the visual impression of lung attenuation mixed with the lower attenuation area representing the abnormal finding. The lower attenuation area is considered less perfused due to decreased pulmonary arterial blood volume or to air trapping and subsequent hypoxic vasoconstriction. Discrimination of mosaic perfusion from ground-glass opacity with adjacent normal lung may sometimes be challenging. Usually, in mosaic perfusion, vessels in the lower attenuation area are smaller than those in higher attenuation area, thus enabling correct diagnosis. With additional expiratory scan at the area in concern is diagnostic in most of the case (8).

Mosaic pattern

Mosaic pattern is often used interchangeably with mosaic perfusion. Because some people use the term mosaic pattern implying the presence of ground-glass opacity adjacent to normal lung, which is misleading, we avoid this usage.

Nodule

A nodule is a focal rounded opacity of any size less than 1cm in diameter. They are usually well-defined in pneumoconiosis but can be ill-defined as is often identified in p-type silicosis (9). Nodule can be used interchangeably with small rounded opacity. A focal rounded opacity more than 1cm in diameter is described as large opacity in this coding system.

Panlobular/multilobular

Panlobular/multilobular is the radiological description of disease processes involving one or more of the secondary lobules in a homogeneous fashion. On CT, the abnormal attenuation area(s) shows homogeneous attenuation and are bounded by interlobular septa.

Parenchymal band (PB)

Parenchymal bands are linear, non-tapering densities 2-5cm in length extending through the lung to contact to pleural surface. Pathologically, parenchymal band represents fibrosis along the bronchovascular sheath or interlobular septa, with distortion of the parenchyma (7). On CT, it is usually identified in the lower lung zones in patients with asbestosis.

Pleural plaque

Pleural plaques, are crater-shaped as well as flat or less elevated thickenings of the pleura with or without calcification and without sub-pleural fibrosis. It is used interchangeably with parietal type pleural thickening.

Pleural thickening

Pleural thickening is visible thickening of the pleura. On CT in normal subjects, this thin strip of soft tissue density is often visible at the interface of the lung and chest wall that represents the combination of pleura, endothoracic fascia and innermost intercostal muscle (10). If any visible thickening of this thin strip is identified, pleural thickening should be described. In this coding system, there are two types of pleural thickening: visceral and parietal type.

Profusion

Profusion is an assessment of the concentration of opacities by the chest radiograph. It is done by comparison with the standard film in ILO system and is regarded as the good indicator intensity of the lung reaction to dust. In this coding system, the term "profusion" is not used and instead "grade" is introduced.

Pseudoplaque

Pseudoplaques are pneumoconiotic nodules often accumulating in the sub-pleural interstitium that mimics or resembles a pleural plaque. In contrast to the smooth appearance in pleural plaque, pseudoplaques show a granular appearance due to the accumulation of small pneumoconiotic nodules in the subpleural pulmonary parenchyma.

Progressive massive fibrosis

Progressive massive fibrosis is characterized by large opacities of pneumoconiotic origin more than 1cm in largest diameter. In silicosis, it is a conglomeration of numbers of silicotic nodules with lung fibrosis. In coal worker's pneumoconiosis, it represents a black mass surrounded by fibrous tissue.

Rounded atelectasis (RA)

Rounded atelectasis is a special type of lung atelectasis, usually seen in association with asbestosis. In most cases, it is the result of pleural fibrosis and adjacent lung collapse; however, in some occasions, it can occur with the development of pleural effusion. The diagnosis is suggested on CT by the combination of the following: wedge-shaped appearance that is usually identified in lower lobes, with convergence of vessels and bronchi from hilum to the mass, the comet tail appearance, the loss of lung volume of the affected lobe, and the presence of diffuse pleural thickening or effusion (11).

Rounded opacity

Rounded opacity is a round-shaped opacity of any etiology. It is synonymous with nodule. It is subcategorized in three groups based on the size; i.e., less than 1.5mm as P, between 1mm and 3mm as Q, and between 3mm and 10mm as R. A round opacity larger than 1cm is designated as large opacity.

Subpleural curvilinear line

Subpleural curvilinear line is a linear opacity within 1cm of the pleura that measures 5-10cm and parallel to the inner chest wall. Usually, it is seen in subjects with asbestosis and the line should persist irrespective of the subject's position either prone or supine. In asbestosis, it represents the early stage of lung fibrosis in the centrilobular areas of the lung (12).

Traction bronchiectasis

Traction bronchiectasis is bronchial dilatation associated with lung organization and fibrosis. It is usually seen in association with ground-glass opacity or consolidation. Principally, it is irreversible but it can be reversible when organization and fibrosis are successfully treated.

Tree-in-bud (TIB)

Tree- in- bud is a reaction to bronchiolar dilatation with filling by mucous, pus and fluid. It resembles a budding tree with branching and indicates the presence of airway disease (13). In pneumoconiosis such as those showing p-type chest radiographs, small rounded opacity can appear as a centrilobular dot or binary structure and can resemble tree-in-bud. However, because the lesion in silicosis is not associated with dilatation of the bronchi, it should not be called tree-in-bud.

References

1. Webb WR, Stern EJ, Kanth N, Gamsu G. Dynamic Pulmonary CT: Findings in Healthy Adult Men. Radiology 1993; 186:117-124
2. Kang EY, Miller RR, M · ler NL. Bronchiectasis: comparison of preoperative thin-section CT and pathologic findings in resected specimens. Radiology 1995; 195:649-654
3. Lynch DA, Newell JD, Tschomper BA, Cink TM, Newman LS, Bethel R. Uncomplicated asthma in adults: comparison of CT appearance of the lungs in asthmatic and healthy subjects. Radiology 1993; 188:829-833
4. Murata K, Itoh H, Todo G, et al. Centrilobular lesions of the lung: demonstration by high-resolution CT and pathologic correlation. Radiology 1986; 161:641-645
5. Snider GL. Pathogenesis and terminology of emphysema. Am J Respir Crit Care Med 1994; 149:1382-1383
6. Heppelston AG. The pathology of honeycomb lung. Thorax 1956; 11:77-93
7. Akira M, Yamamoto S, Yokoyama K, et al. Asbestosis: high-resolution CT-pathologic correlation. Radiology 1990; 176:389-394
8. Arakawa H, Webb WR, McCowin M, Katsou G, Lee KN, Seitz RF. Inhomogeneous lung attenuation at thin-section CT: diagnostic value of expiratory scans. Radiology 1998; 206:89-94
9. Akira M, Higashihara T, Yokoyama K, et al. Radiographic type p pneumoconiosis: high-resolution CT. Radiology 1989; 171:117-123
10. Im JG, Webb WR, Rosen A, Gamsu G. Costal pleura: appearances at high-resolution CT. Radiology 1989; 171:125-131
11. Lynch DA, Gamsu G, Ray CS, Aberle DR. Asbestos-related focal lung masses: manifestations on conventional and high-resolution CT scans. Radiology 1988; 169:603-607

12. Yoshimura H, Hatakeyama M, Otsuji H, et al. Pulmonary asbestosis: CT study of subpleural curvilinear shadow. Work in progress. Radiology 1986; 158:653-658
13. Aquino SL, Gamsu G, Webb WR, Kee ST. Tree-in-bud pattern: frequency and significance on thin section CT. J Comput Assist Tomogr 1996; 20:594-599

Chapter 2 Coding CT-Classification in Occupational and Environmental Respiratory Disease (OERD)

Kurt G. Hering[1] and Thomas Kraus[2]

[1]Department of Diagnostic Radiology, Radiooncology and Neclear Medicine, Radiologische Klinik, Knappschaftskrankenhaus, Dortmund, Wiecksweg 27, 44309 Dortmund, Germany

[2]Institute and Outpatient Clinic for Occupational Medicine, University Hospital Aachen, Pauwelsstr. 30, D-52074 Aachen, Germany

Foreword

The coding system is to be applied as strictly descriptive system and is not diagnostic. It is intended to cover all aspects of occupational and environmental disorders dealing with parenchymal and pleural abnormalities. Although some of the descriptive terms are classically associated with pneumoconiosis{xe "pneumoconiosis"}, for example rounded opacities{xe "rounded opacities"} with silicosis{xe "silicosis"}, or interlobular septal and intralobular non-septal lines and honeycombing with asbestosis{xe "asbestosis"}, these are radiographic patterns that must be carefully considered for an appropriate differential diagnosis reached.

In this coding system neither reference films{xe "reference films"} nor text have precedence over each other. To successfully classify an HRCT study the reader needs to use both text and reference films. For detailed explanation of the terms the reader is referred to chapter 1 on glossary of terms.

For screening{xe "screening"} purposes 6 to 8 slices are taken, distributed over all zones, preferably in the prone{xe "prone"} position. The reading sheet{xe "reading sheet"} has correspondence for each zone. If more than one slice per zone is taken, all findings per zone have to be summarized and classified for each zone{xe "zone"}. See reading sheet{xe "reading sheet"} example (Fig. 2.1).

The “Comments/Summary” Section leaves the opportunity for free text.

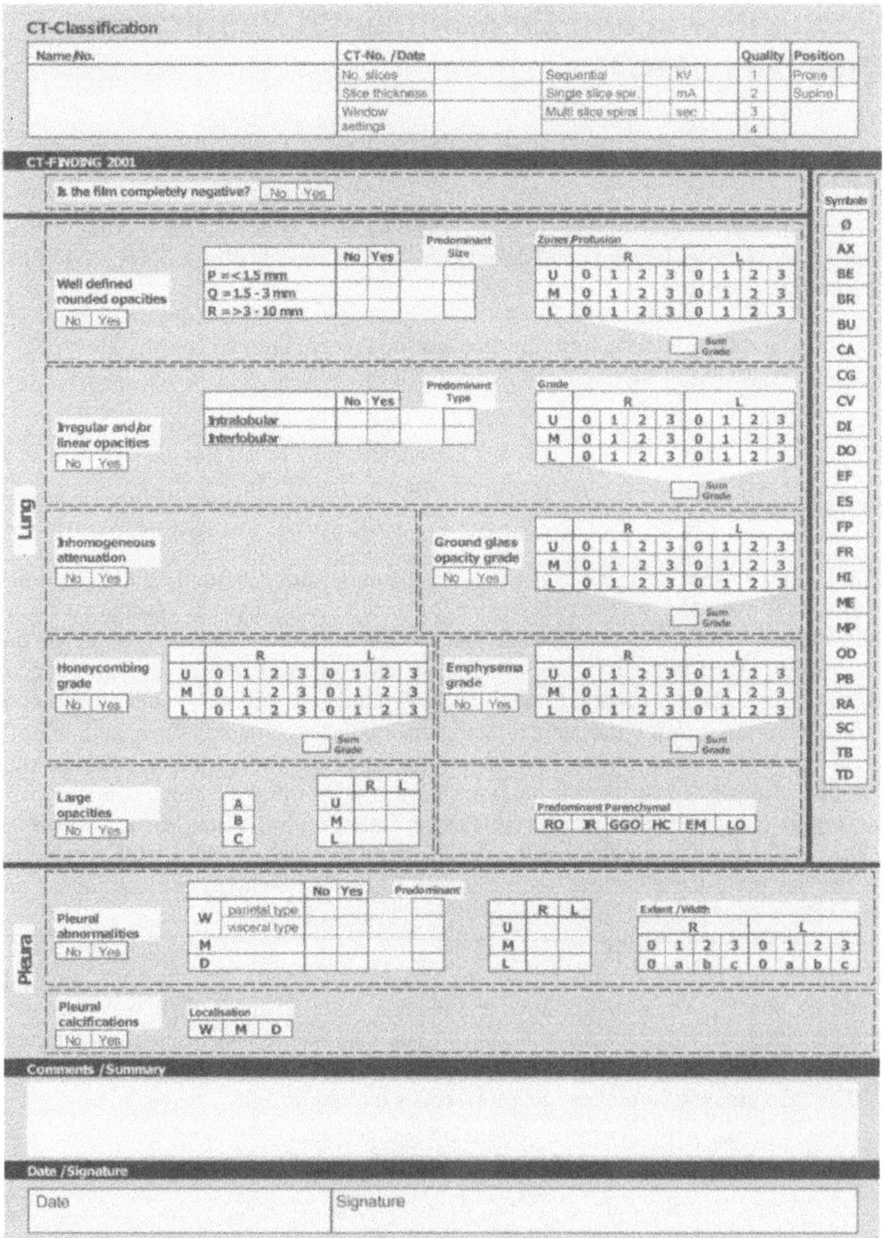

CT-Classification

Name/No.	CT-No. /Date						Quality		Position	
	No. slices		Sequential		kV		1		Prone	
	Slice thickness		Single slice spir.		mA		2		Supine	
	Window settings		Multi slice spiral		sec		3			
							4			

CT-FINDING 2001

Is the film completely negative? No Yes

Symbols: Ø, AX, BE, BR, BU, CA, CG, CV, DI, DO, EF, ES, FP, FR, HI, ME, MP, OD, PB, RA, SC, TB, TD

Lung

Well defined rounded opacities — No Yes

	No	Yes	Predominant Size
P = < 1.5 mm			
Q = 1.5 - 3 mm			
R = > 3 - 10 mm			

Zones/Profusion

	R				L			
U	0	1	2	3	0	1	2	3
M	0	1	2	3	0	1	2	3
L	0	1	2	3	0	1	2	3

Sum Grade

Irregular and/or linear opacities — No Yes

	No	Yes	Predominant Type
Intralobular			
Interlobular			

Grade

	R				L			
U	0	1	2	3	0	1	2	3
M	0	1	2	3	0	1	2	3
L	0	1	2	3	0	1	2	3

Sum Grade

Inhomogeneous attenuation — No Yes

Ground glass opacity grade — No Yes

	R				L			
U	0	1	2	3	0	1	2	3
M	0	1	2	3	0	1	2	3
L	0	1	2	3	0	1	2	3

Sum Grade

Honeycombing grade — No Yes

	R				L			
U	0	1	2	3	0	1	2	3
M	0	1	2	3	0	1	2	3
L	0	1	2	3	0	1	2	3

Sum Grade

Emphysema grade — No Yes

	R				L			
U	0	1	2	3	0	1	2	3
M	0	1	2	3	0	1	2	3
L	0	1	2	3	0	1	2	3

Sum Grade

Large opacities — No Yes

A / B / C

	R	L
U		
M		
L		

Predominant Parenchymal: RO IR GGO HC EM LO

Pleura

Pleural abnormalities — No Yes

		No	Yes	Predominant
W	parietal type			
	visceral type			
M				
D				

	R	L
U		
M		
L		

Extent / Width

R				L			
0	1	2	3	0	1	2	3
0	a	b	c	0	a	b	c

Pleural calcifications — No Yes

Localisation: W M D

Comments / Summary

Date / Signature

Date	Signature

Fig. 2.1 Reading Sheet

Basic Data

Name/No.:
Data for Registration:
CT-Information:
- Date and Number
- Modality
  - Sequential CT{xe "CT:Sequential"}
  - Spiral-Single-Slice CT{xe "CT:Spiral-Single-Slice"}
  - Spiral-Multi-Slice CT{xe "CT:Spiral-Multi-Slice"}
- No. of slices for evaluation – at least 6 reference-slices
- Slice thickness{xe "Slice thickness"} – 1-2 mm
- Window settings – preferably 2 window settings
- Quality{xe "Quality"}:

  1 = good; 2 = acceptable, with no technical defect likely to impair classification; 3 = acceptable, with some technical defect but still adequate for classification purposes; 4 = unreadable
- Position –preferably prone position at least for the 6 reference slices

The Initial or Basic question

"Is the film completely negative?"
If "Yes" just fill date and signature at the bottom of the sheet; if "No" the classification has to be done step by step for each item!

Well defined rounded opacities

Absence (No) or Presence (Yes) has to be reported.

It includes all measurable, well defined rounded opacities{xe "rounded opacities"} from <1.5 mm in diameter (= P{xe "P"}), between 1.5 and 3 mm (= Q{xe "Q"}), to 3 up to 10 mm (= R{xe "R"}).
NOTE: It has to be remembered that hardcopy CT images are diminished and the dimensions of opacities recorded should be true or life size measurements.

The overall distribution is recorded in a grading{xe "grading"} system, regardless of form and size, for each side right (R) or left (L) and each zone of the thorax: upper (U) – arch of the aorta{xe "arch of the aorta"} and above, middle (M) – arch of the aorta down to the inferior pulmonary vein{xe "inferior pulmonary vein"}, lower (L) – inferior pulmonary vein and below including diaphragm{xe "diaphragm"}. The precise definition of the borderline of the zone is not crucial for the application of the system.

0 = no definitive opacities
1 = mild, small opacities definitely present but few in number
2 = moderate, numerous small opacities
3 = severe, small opacities very numerous, normal anatomical lung structures poorly visible

It is possible to check more than one opacity, e.g. P and Q or another combination, and then the predominant size P, Q or R has to be recorded.

Sum of grading, regardless of size, side and zone.
Possible ranging from 0 to 18.

e.g.	R –	U – 3	L –	U – 2	
		M – 2		M – 1	
		L – 0		L – 0	Sum = 8

Irregular and/or linear opacities

Absence (No) or Presence (Yes) has to be reported.

Morphologic abnormalities of parenchymal disease: Intralobular opacities,
Interlobular opacities

Intralobular opacities include dotlike lesions in early asbestosis or hypersensitivity pneumonitis. Subpleural curvilinear opacities are a specific distribution of fibrotic intralobular core structures, paralleling the pleura, few millimetres or less in thickness and usually 1 cm from the pleural surface and are reported as a symbol ("SC"). Parenchymal bands are peripheral linear opacities, branching from the surface of a thickened pleura. They have to be reported with pleural abnormalities separately as a symbol ("PB"). If there is no visible contact to the pleural surface (maybe due to limited number of slices) they should be mentioned as translobular bands and additional explanatory notes should be made without using a symbol.

Mark the absence (X) or presence (X) for each item and predominant type.

The overall distribution is recorded in a grading system, regardless of type, for each side right (R) or left (L) and each zone, upper (U), middle (M) and lower (L):

0 = no definite abnormalities
1 = mild, abnormalities definitely present but few in number
2 = moderate, numerous abnormalities
3 = severe, abnormalities very numerous, normal anatomical lung structures poorly visible

Sum of grading, regardless of type, side and zone.
Possible ranging from 0 to 18.

e.g.	R –	U – 0	L –	U – 0	
		M – 2		M – 1	
		L – 2		L – 2	Sum = 7

Additional parenchymal abnormalities

Inhomogeneous attenuation:
Absence (No) or Presence (Yes) has to be reported.

Inhomogeneity is possibly due to mosaic perfusion (MP) or ground glass opacity (GGO). In cases where GGO is present, grading has to be done for each side and each zone by judging the extent of the finding:

1 = focal
2 = patchy
3 = diffuse

In a case of mosaic perfusion related to air trapping or vessel obstruction, use only the symbol "MP".

Honeycombing (HC):
Honeycombing can occur with and without GGO. Absence (No) or Presence (Yes) has to be reported. Irregular opacities within the HC-area are not classified separately.
Grading has to be done for each side and each zone:

1 = mild, up to 10 mm in the subpleural parenchyma
2 = moderate; >10 to 30 mm in the subpleural parenchyma
3 = severe; >30 mm up to whole area of one zone

Emphysema:
Presence (Yes) or absence (No) has to be reported.

Emphysema is graded for right and left side and for all zones.

1 = mild, up to 15 % of the area of one zone
2 = moderate, between 15 and 30%
3 = severe, > 30 %

Differentiation - e.g. acinar, panlobular, subpleural or cicatricial - must be given as a comment. If bullae are present, the symbol "BU" has to be noted.
NOTE: An overall sum of grading for both sides and all zones is required for GGO, Emphysema or Honeycombing.

Large opacities

Absence (No) or Presence (Yes) has to be reported.

Pneumoconiotic as well as non-pneumoconiotic opacities larger than 1 cm in diameter have to be reported. Rounded atelectasis (“RA”) is not reported as a large opacity. Usually in case of “RA” there is a definite connection to pleural thickening and this has to be recorded as “Visceral Type” with the symbol “RA”.

Opacities are measured in 2 perpendicular axes, as soon as the mean diameter is >1 cm. All large opacities of both sides are combined. Additional symbols can be used, e.g. suspicious for carcinoma = symbol "CA"; for pneumonia = symbol "OD" with additional text.

A = One or more opacities, extent >1 cm up to 1/4 of the area (quadrant) of the right side of the CT-slice at the carina (see Fig. 2.2)

B = Area of one or sum of more opacities larger than „A“, less than 1/2 of the area (2 quadrants) of the right side of the CT-slice at the carina

C = Area of one or sum of more opacities larger than half of the area of the right side of the CT-slice at the carina

Predominance

Reach a conclusion regarding the predominant finding from the recorded signs:

RO (Rounded opacities) IR (Irregular/linear opacities)
GGO (Ground glass opacities) HC (Honeycombing)
EM (Emphysema) LO (Large opacities)

If there are two or more findings in equal predominance, check each of them and give a comment!

Pleural abnormalities

Two types are differentiated according to the CT appearance: Parietal and Visceral type. Absence (No) or Presence (Yes) has to be reported.

The term “Parietal Type” includes the typical tableland-shape as well as the flat (less elevated) thickening of the pleura without subpleural fibrosis. For classifying there should be no lower limit. If detectable and measurable, it should be reported.

“Visceral Type” is often described as “Diffuse Pleural Thickening” and is always associated with the presence of subpleural fibrosis or parenchymal bands and rounded atelectasis. Additional information is obligatory when a visceral type is reported as pleural abnormality, either irregular and linear opacities or symbols like “PB” or “RA”.

At first report the presence (X) or absence (X) for each item, location and predominant type, secondly document the distribution of both types combined for right and left and for each zone!

Extent and Width are reported independently for each side, but again for both types combined.

Extent:

All abnormalities of the wall and mediastinum except the findings at the diaphragm are measured. Choose the slice with the most extensive pleural thickening for each zone and transfer and add it (virtually) to the slice, positioned at the carina (see drawing, Fig. 2.2). Extent is measured in terms of degrees of the circumference of 360° for each side:

1 = up to 90° (< ¼)
2 = > 90° up to 180° (¼ – ½)
3 = > 180° (> ½)

Width:

The thickest part of the parietal or the visceral type of the 3 chosen slices will be measured:

a = up to 5 mm
b = 5 – 10 mm
c = > 10 mm

Pleural abnormalities of the Mediastinum ("M") and the diaphragm ("D") will be documented as absent (X) or present (X).

Findings at the diaphragm are not measured concerning extent and width.

Pleural calcifications:

Absence (No) or Presence (Yes) has to be reported.
If present, localisation has to be reported for wall (W), mediastinum (M) and diaphragm (D). Per definition the paravertebral space belongs to the wall.

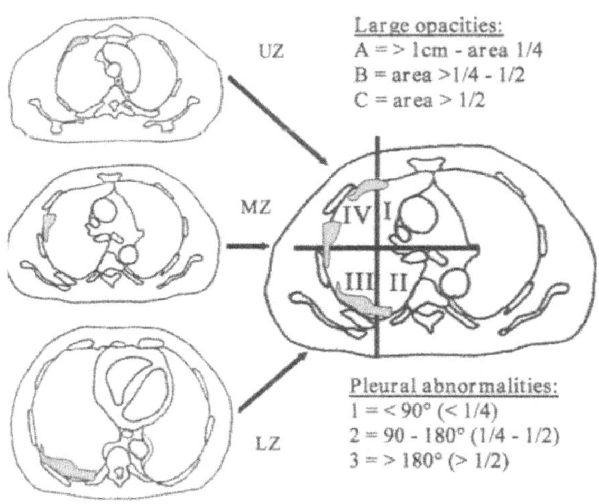

Fig. 2.2. Measurement of Large Opacities and Extent of Pleural Thickening

Symbols

Symbols describe additional features related to dust exposure and other etiologies. The definitions of symbols assume a qualifying phrase such as “changes indicative of” or “compatible with” (Table 2.1).

Use capital letters to differentiate between ILO-symbols (used for the classification) and CT-symbols.

Table 2.1.

Symbol	Definition
0	None
AX	Coalescence of small pneumoconiotic opacities
BE	Bronchiectasis; all types, including traction bronchiectasis
BR	Bronchial wall thickening
BU	Bullae, additional information on emphysema
CA	Lung Cancer
CG	Calcified Granuloma
CV	Cavity, central necrosis, liquid and/or air containing
DI	Distortion of intrathoracic structures and organs
DO	Dependent Opacity
EF	Effusion, free or loculated pleural fluid
ES	Eggshell calcification of hilar and/or mediastinal lymph nodes
FP	Fat Pad, extrapleural/subcostal fat
FR	Fractured Rib (s)
HI	Enlargement of hilar and/or mediastinal lymph nodes, >1,5-2 cm
ME	Malignant Mesothelioma of the pleura, the pericardium or the peritoneum
MP	Mosaic Perfusion
OD	Other Disease; comments under „Additional Findings“
PB	Parenchymal Band, due to pleuroparenchymal scars
RA	Rounded Atelectasis
SC	Subpleural curvilinear lines
TB	Tuberculosis
TD	Tree in Bud

Comments/Summary

Comments

Additional information on each paragraph can be documented. If there are findings which are not covered by the evaluation sheet, e.g. descriptive terms for particular patterns of intralobular opacities, they can be mentioned in this section of the Reading Sheet (Fig. 2.1).

Summary

A conclusive summary is necessary, e.g. findings are compatible with occupational or non-occupational disease, differential diagnostic considerations should be mentioned.

References

Al Jarad N, Wilkinson P, Pearson MC, Rudd RM (1992) A new high resolution computed tomography scoring system for pulmonary fibrosis, pleural disease and emphysema in patients with asbestos related disease. Br J Ind Med 49:73-84

Hering KG (1991) Auswertung und Einordnung von CT-Befunden bei berufsbedingten Lungen- und Pleuraveränderungen in Anlehnung and die ILO-Staublungen-Klassifikation. Röntgenpraxis 45:304-308

Hering KG, Tuengerthal S, Kraus T (2004) Standardisierte CT/HRCT-Klassifikation der Bundesrepublik Deutschland für arbeits-und um-weltbedingte Thoraxerkrankungen. Der Radiologe 5:500-511

Huuskonen O, Kivisaari L, Zitting A, Taskinen K, Tossavainen A, Vehmas T (2001) High resolution computed tomography classification of lung fibrosis for patients with asbestos related disease. Scand J Work Environ Health 27:106-112

Kraus T, Raithel HJ, Hering KG (1996) Evaluation and classification of high- resolution computed tomographic findings in patients with pneumoconiosis. Int Arch Occup Environ Health 68:249-254

Suganuma N, Kusska Y, Hosoda Y, Shida H, Morikubo H, Nakajima Y, Akira M, Matsumoto T, Hiraga Y (2001) The Japanese Classification of Computed Tomography for Pneumoconiosis with Standard Films. Comparison with the ILO International Classification of Radiographs for Pneumoconioses. J Occup Health 43:24-31

Webb WR, Müller NL, Naidich DP (2000) High-Resolution CT of the lung, 3rd Edition, Lippincott-Raven, Philadelphia, New York

Chapter 3 Technical Aspects and Imaging Parameters in HRCT

Tapio Vehmas[1] and Leena Kivisaari[2]

[1]Finnish Institute of Occupational Health, Topeliuksenkatu 41 a A, FIN-00250 Helsinki, Finland

[2]Department of Radiology, Helsinki University Central Hospital, Haartmaninkatu 4, P.O. Box 380, FIN-00029 Helsinki, Finland

Introduction

Despite the fast technical development of magnetic resonance imaging, computed tomography (CT) is still the most accurate imaging modality to show the anatomical detail in such aerated organs as the lungs. By modern slip-ring technology, spiral CT, capable to produce thin section images (1-2 mm) with high or ultra high algorithm (high resolution CT, HRCT), has become available on practically all types of scanners. Spiral CT, in either one or multirow form, is a volume scanning procedure in non-planar geometry, data acquisition extending over selected amount of rotations

The technical quality of the scanner, patient characteristics (especially the size of the body part to be imaged) and some other technical variables, such as the development process of the hard copies, may influence the selection of imaging parameters. From the epidemiological and research point of view, the imaging parameters are best standardized to make all images in the study comparable with each other. The reading sheet (Chapter 2, Fig. 2.1) has space for the description of these parameters. At least any deviations from the agreed protocol (Nikko Agreement, Table 3.1) should be described.

The differences in performance of scanners are mostly in the power of the x-ray system and of the computer. The power of x-ray system creates the limits for scanning times and volumes. Multislice CT performs from two to sixteen slices in a single rotation. The method is faster than single slice CT and reduces artifacts produced by patient moving. The x-ray tube heating, constraining parameters in single-slice scanning is reduced in multislice scanning.

To minimize motion artifacts, the scanner should be able to produce short exposure times, preferably less than 1 second. Thin section slices computed by ultra high algorithm may be generated from the raw data produced with equipment capable for volume CT, spiral or the most recent technical approach, multirow or multislice CT (Anonymous 2002). This has the advantage of no extra radiation and of an exposure in short time (0.5 sec) added to the spiral imaging (Kalender et al. 2000).

Spatial and contrast resolution along the z axis, previously a limiting step for slice images, has improved because of the possibility of reconstructing arbitrarily many images in any direction and any slice thickness for the scanned volume (Kalender et al. 2000).

Unfortunately, there are several parameters to be optimized in HRCT and relatively few scientific studies supporting their adequate use.

Patient posture

It is widely accepted that imaging should normally be done at full inspiration to prevent false positive findings resulting from poor lung aeration. The demonstration of air trapping may need expiratory scans (Webb 1997). The standard scanning direction is axial although special directions have been reported in special indications (Uchisako et al. 1997). Scanning with the patient in prone position (Murray et al. 1995) has the advantage that dorsal parts of the lungs, i.e. the region where most fibrotic changes in asbestosis are located, will be free of dependent oedema and possible hypoventilation. Obese patients may find the prone lie difficult and full inspiration may thus be prevented. Supine lie may then be used. Supine imaging only may be used in silicosis cases (Zhang et al. 1995).

Exposure parameters

The question of slice thickness is closely related to whether the patient should be imaged with HRCT of conventional or volume CT. According to Gevenois et al. (1994) asbestosis diagnosis was best made and parenchymal bands best visualised with HRCT while pleural lesions were best detected with conventional CT. Both of them may be calculated separately and retrospectively from an acquired data volume performed by spiral/multislice CT. It is the general custom to use HRCT for a detailed view of lung pathology.

In HRCT, scanning with the thinnest possible collimation (from less than 1 to 2 mm) has been recommended (Webb et al. 1996) to keep the spatial resolution (sharpness of the image) optimal and the noise (random variation of the CT number, mainly dominated by the finite number of detected x-rays) as low as possible (Judy 2000). The best visualisation of nodules of 1-5 mm in size was found with 3 mm spiral slices when compared to 1mm, 5 mm or 8 mm slices (Paranjpe & Bergin 1994). They found it difficult to separate between vessels and nodules in 1-mm slices. The difference between 1.5 and 3 mm slices was minimal in the study by Murata et al. (1988) in such lesions as lymphangitic carcinomatosis and radiation fibrosis. The personal experience of the authors is that there was little if any difference in image quality between 1 and 2 mm slices when lungs were studied after transplantation (Ikonen et al 1997). 2 mm thick conventional and helical slices with pitches 1.0, 1.5 and 2.0 were graded equivalent to 1.0 mm HRCT slices when animal lungs were studied (Hopper et al. 1998). Due to the simultaneous increase in voxel size and collimation the noise varies inversely with the square root of collimation (Paranjpe & Bergin 1994). Increasing the radiation load (mAs) may counteract this. As far as we know, no one has suggested lung imaging with slices thinner as 1 mm. By multislice computed tomography (volume scanning) it is possible to calculate any slice thickness or image manipulation effect from the acquired data volume, making the importance of separately acquired HRCT to be less prominent.

For simplicity and for radiation protection purposes, it would be ideal to have a limited number of HRCT slices. This is possible if the disease under observation is homogeneously distributed in lungs. A single prone scan showed a relatively high accuracy in asbestos-related lung disease (Murray et al. 1995). Three-level thin section CT revealed the pathologic changes associated with idiopathic pulmonary fibrosis as well as sections at 10-mm intervals (Kazeeroni et al. 1997). Overall emphysema could be quantified by using only three slices: one in the upper, middle, and lower lung (Hitsuda et al. 2000). Diseases with non-homogenous distribution (pleural changes, bronchiectases, and few nodules) may fail to manifest in such a short protocol. The Nikko Agreement (Table 3.1) tries to compromise between the high radiation exposure associated with a liberal number of slices and the possible false negative findings due to too few slices.

While the voltage is best set as recommended by the manufacturer of the equipment the selection of current (mA) has a profound effect on the image quality and radiation exposure, which are inversely proportional to each other. Majurin et al. (1994) studied the ability of slices with 1-mm collimation to show asbestos-related pathology by changing the tube current. 160 mAs slices gave good images in most entities while using 120 mAs led to poorer visibility of subpleural short lines. 60 mAs images showed inferiority in most studied findings. Their findings concerning lungs after radiotherapy are similar (Majurin et al. 1995). Zwirewich et al. (1991) compared the diagnostic potential of HRCT at 20 and 200 mA (1,5 mm collimation, 2 s rotation time and 120 kV). The low-dose method was equal in the evaluation of vessels, bronchi, the anatomy of secondary pulmonary lobules, the characterisation of reticulation, honeycomb cysts and interlobular septa. It failed to demonstrate ground glass opacities and emphysema in a few cases and showed more linear streak artifacts. It is possible that the newer generation CT equipment may operate with less current, even be automatically modulated according to anatomical structures, still maintaining the image quality (Kalender et al. 2000). The author (TV) uses 100 mAs for HRCT in pneumoconioses. Multislice CT has a potential to increase the radiation dose of the patients. Radiation exposure is dealt with in a separate section.

Imaging parameters

The window level (WL, expressed in Hounsfield units, HU) governs the brightness of the image while the window width (WW, as above) sets the contrast. If narrow windows are used to study the hard copies, separate printouts for lung and mediastinum /soft tissues are needed. Suganuma et al. (unpublished) compared the visibility of rounded, linear and reticular opacities by using the lung window (WL -650 / WW 1200) and a single wide window (WL -400/ WW 2000). They found the lung window significantly better considering small rounded opacities, septal /non-septal lines, ground glass opacity and emphysema. A wide window dilutes subtle differences in lung density but may show the pleuroparenchymal findings (visceral pleural / diffuse fibrosis) better. A low window mean (-800 to -900 HU) is needed for the optimal visualisation of emphysema (Webb et al. 1996). The selection of the window is also related to the particular equipment used, including the workstation monitor and the hard copy processing device. In filmless image reading, more attention should be paid to the brightness and the contrast of the monitor. There should be either a proper standardisation of the monitor contrast and brightness based on phantom images or a creation of special criteria for anatomic structures, which should be visible in the images of the normal lung. Without such system, the image quality may be evaluated in a matter similar to the ILO 1980 classification: 1 = good; 2 = acceptable, with no technical defect likely to impair classification; 3 = acceptable, with some technical defect but still adequate for classification purposes; 4 = unreadable. An independent observer best assesses the image quality, but this is seldom practically possible. The authors' recommendations for the selection of the window level and width are given in Table 3.1.

The larger the image matrix the more detailed the images will be. To our knowledge, the HRCT hard-copy size has not been studied regarding diagnostic performance. Schaefer et al. (1992) studied a large material of digital chest radiographs with full-size images and those reduced to 67 %, 50 % and 45 % in length. Their detection of micronodular opacities and lines deteriorated with declining image size. On the other hand, in their smaller material van Heesewijk et al. (1997) could not find a difference in radiologists' performance in detecting pulmonary, mediastinal or pleural pathology between life-size or minified films. It seems that care is needed not to loose small details in HRCT with too reduced image size. These problems are going to be less prominent in filmless image reading on the monitor.

The authors of this book have discussed the imaging parameters and give their consensus recommendation (Nikko Agreement) in Table 3.1.

Table 3.1. Nikko Agreement on imaging parameters. The images should be exposed at full inspiration and the high resolution algorithm should be used

Parameter	Comment	Clarification
Slice thickness	1 – 2 mm	
Number of slices	Minimum 6	Carina 1, above it 1, below it 4
Scan time	< 1 second	
kV	120 – 150	
mAs	40 – 100 (up to 150)	
Patient position	Prone	
Image windowing	Lung and mediastinal windows normally	Lung: WL -400 – -700 HU WW 1200 – 2000 HU Mediastinal: WL 20 – 50 HU WW 300 – 500 HU
	(If a single window is used)	Single: WL -400 HU WW 2000 HU
Matrix size	≥512 pixels	
No. of images	≤12 in a 35 x 43 cm film	Image size ≥ 10 x 10 cm

References

Anonymous (2002) Evaluation. Multislice computed tomography systems. Health Devices 31; 161-88

Hitsuda Y, Kawasaki Y, Igishi T, Yasuda K, Kato K, Matsumoto S, Nakamoto M, Hashimoto K, Fujii Y, Miyata M, Sasaki T, Shimizu E (2000) A study of the minimum number of slices required for quantification of pulmonary emphysema by computed tomography. Nihon Kokyuki Gakkai Zasshi 38; 430-6

Hopper KD, Kasales CJ, Wise SW, TenHave TR, Hills JR, Mahraj RM, Wilson RP, Weaver JS (1998) The optimization of helical thoracic CT. J Comput Assist Tomogr. 22; 418-24

Ikonen T, Kivisaari L, Taskinen E, Uusitalo M, Aarnio P, Harjula A (1997) Acute rejection diagnosed with CT in a porcine experimental lung transplantation model. Scand Cardiovasc J 31;25-32

Judy PF (2000) CT image quality and parameters affecting the CT image. In: Goldman LW, Fowlkes JB (ed.) Categorial course in diagnostic radiology physics: CT and US cross-sectional imaging, pp117-125

Kalender W, Fuchs TOJ (2000) Principles and performance of single- and multislice spiral CT. In: Goldman LW, Fowlkes JB (ed.) Categorial course of diagnostic radiology physics: CT and US cross-sectional imaging, pp 127-142

Kazeeroni AE, Martinez FJ, Flint A, Jamadar DA, Gross BH, Spizarny DL, Cascade PN, Whyte RI, Lynch JP 3rd, Toews G(1997) Thin-section CT obtained at 10-mm increments versus limited three-level thin-section CT for idiopathic pulmonary fibrosis: correlation with pathologic scoring. AJR 169; 977-83

Majurin ML, Valavaara R, Varpula M, Kurki T, Kulmala J (1995) Low-dose and conventional-dose high resolution CT of pulmonary changes in breast cancer patients treated by tangential field therapy. Eur J Radiol 20; 114-9

Majurin M-L, Varpula M, Kurki T, Pakkala L (1994) High-resolution CT of the lung in asbestos-exposed subjects. Comparison of low-dose and high-dose HRCT. Acta Radiol 35; 473-7

Murata K, Khan A, Rojas KA, Herman PG (1988) Optimization of computed tomography technique to demonstrate the fine structure of the lung. Invest Radiol 23; 170-5

Murray KA, Gamsu G, Webb WR, Salmon CJ, Egger MJ (1995) High-resolution computed tomography sampling for detection of asbestos-related lung disease. Acad Radiol 2, 111-5

Paranjpe DV, Bergin CJ (1994) Spiral CT of the lungs: Optimal technique and resolution compared with conventional CT. AJR 162; 561-7

Uchisako H, Matsumoto T, Kuramitsu T, Tamaka N, Miura G, Nakamura H, Matsunaga N (1997) Thin-section oblique CT with 25 degrees cranially tilted images. Evaluation of tumors adjacent to the interlobar fissures. Acta Radiol 38; 246-9

Webb WR (1997) Radiology of obstructive pulmonary disease. AJR 169; 637-47

Webb WR, Müller NL, Naidich DP (1996) High-resolution CT of the lung. Lippincott-Raven Publishers (2nd ed.), Philadelphia-New York

Zhang X, Kusaka Y, Ishii Y (1995) Computed tomography of pneumoconiosis (in Japanese). Sangyo Eiseigaku Zasshi 37; 321-8

Zwirewich CV, Mayo JR, Muller NL (1991) Low-dose high-resolution CT of lung parenchyma. Radiology 180; 413-7

Part II

Practice and Study Protocol

Chapter 4 Radiation Exposure and Risk Assessment in HRCT

Kanae Nishizawa[1], Shinji Yoshinaga[1], Juhani Karppinen[2], and Tapio Vehmas[3]

[1]National Institute of Radiological Sciences, 4-9-1Anagawa, Inage-ku, Chiba 263-8555, Japan

[2]Radiation and Nuclear Safety Authority, P.O. Box 14, FIN-00881 Helsinki, Finland

[3]Finnish Institute of Occupational Health, Topeliuksenkatu 41 aA, FIN 00250 Helsinki, Finland

Introduction

CT is a widely employed modality and delivers a considerable part of the total collective dose in radiology. The use of CT examinations has continued to increase in recent years in spite of the widespread availability of MR imaging. In view of the newest technical developments in CT, it is not expected that this trend will reverse in the foreseeable future. On the contrary, the possibilities of the multi-slice spiral CT will most likely lead to a further increase in the number of CT examinations performed.

The International Commission on Radiological Protection (ICRP) recommended that the application of the dose limits to medical exposure is not appropriate, because the examinations are usually intended to provide a direct benefit to the exposed individual. Nevertheless, from the safety point of view, exposure due to radiological examination must be kept minimal, while sufficient image quality be maintained. This is known as the ALARA (as low as reasonably achievable) principle (ICRP, 1996). This is especially true in the screening, since most examinees are supposed to be healthy. Risk-benefit of every screening should be evaluated.

The European Commission (EC 1999) has developed recommendations concerning achievable standards of good practice in high resolution CT (HRCT) of the chest. The subjective image criteria include critical reproduction of anatomical features. Criteria concerning patient dose are given in special measurable quantities associated with the examination technique used for dosimetric phantoms. In clinical imaging, the quality of diagnostic information and the radiation exposure must always be weighted against each other.

The conditions of exposure in CT, in which thin slices of the patient are irradiated in rotational geometry by a fan beam of x-rays, are quite different from those in conventional x-ray examinations. Specific dosimetric techniques are therefore needed to assess patient doses and risks and to allow monitoring for different types of CT examinations. In this chapter, possible doses from HRCT screening will be evaluated on the basis of actual measurement data, and then risk-benefit of HRCT screening will be discussed.

Dose evaluation

Two methods have been widely used in the estimation of the effective dose or the risk from CT examination; the estimation in terms of computed tomography dose index (CTDI) and the measurement with an anthropomorphic tissue equivalent phantom. The CTDI is well defined and its calculation protocol is well documented internationally as described in the following chapters. However, some of simplified assumption is necessary for the evaluation of the effective dose of patients. The method based on the measurement with an anthropomorphic phantom is in close accordance with the evaluation method recommended by ICRP. Its shortcoming is that the estimation is valid for a particular anthropomorphic phantom and is not applicable to all physiques. These two methods have merits and demerits and are complementary; it is useful for an average risk evaluation.

Dose quantities

The dosimetric quantity widely used in CT is the ***computed tomography dose index, CTDI*** (Shope, 1981, FDA,1984). The CT dose index, given in units of mGy, is defined as:

$$\text{CTDI} = \frac{1}{N \cdot T} \int_{-\infty}^{+\infty} D_1(z)dz \,.$$

Here $D_1(z)$ is the dose profile for a single slice per rotation along a line perpendicular to the tomographic plane, where dose is measured as absorbed dose to air. N is the number of tomographic sections produced in a single 360° rotation of the x-ray tube. T is the nominal tomographic section thickness. The traditional CTDI is integrated from -7 T to +7 T as defined by the FDA (1984).

In practice, the dosimetry in CT is based on measurements of the line integral of the dose profile. Such measurements may be accomplished using a stack of thermo-luminescent dosimeters (TLDs) or, more conveniently, using an appropriately calibrated 100 mm long pencil-shaped ionisation chamber. The output of the chamber represents the CT dose of a single slice. When the active length L of the chamber is multiplied by this dose D_1, the resulting product of dose and length, $D_1 \cdot L$, is equivalent to the area under the dose profile.

Reference values for CT are based on measurements in a standard CT dosimetry phantom (FDA, 1984). Standard head or body phantoms are presently homogeneous cylinders of polymethylmethacrylate (PMMA), with diameters of

16 cm or 32 cm. A weighted sum $CTDI_w$ of CTDI values measured at the centre and 10 mm below the surface of standard CT head and body dosimetry phantoms provide more relevant information from the average dose to patient's tissue (EC, 1999, IEC 2001)):

$$CTDI_w = 1/3\ CTDI_{100}\ (\text{centre}) + 2/3\ CTDI_{100}\ (\text{peripheral}).$$

According to an international standard (IEC, 2001), the $CTDI_w$ should be displayed on the operator's console; if the total thickness of slices produced in one scan is not equal to the table increment per rotation, a corrected $CTDI_w$ value should be displayed on the operator's console describing the average dose over the total volume scanned for the selected conditions of operation.

Since clinical studies seldom consist of one scan, the total dose in the procedure is calculated as a sum over all contributing scans, because tissues irradiated in one slice receive contributions from other slices due to scattering and field overlap. If the table feed (Δd) per rotation differs from the slice thickness (N·T), an average dose quantity, the ***multiple scan average dose (MSAD)*** takes into account the distance between successive slices (rotations) and represents the average dose at the scanning area.

$$\text{MSAD} = \frac{1}{\Delta d}\int_{-L/2}^{L/2} D_1(z)dz = \frac{1}{\Delta d}(D_1 \cdot L) = \text{CTDI}/(\Delta d / N \cdot T),$$

where Δd /N·T is called the pitch (table feed Δd per rotation relative to N·T).

Typical multiple-scan average doses are in the range of 40-60 mGy for head scans and 10-40 mGy for body scans (EC, 1999).

In CT examinations, the analogic quantity of the dose area product (DAP) is the ***dose length product (DLP)***. The DLP, given in units of mGycm, can be estimated from an integral of the multiple-scan dose profile D(z) for the sequence (examination)

$$\text{DLP} = \int_{-\infty}^{+\infty} D(z)dz\ .$$

When CT examination consists of many scans (or rotations), DLP is simply the product of the DLP_1 of one scan (or one rotation in helical scanning) and the number of scans n (or rotations)

$$\text{DLP} = n \int_{-L/2}^{L/2} D_1(z)dz = n \cdot DLP_1 = n \cdot \Delta d \cdot \text{MSAD}$$
$$= n \cdot N \cdot T \cdot \text{CTDI}.$$

Therefore, DLP per sequence is the product of the table scan length n·Δd and the average dose MSAD or the product of the number of scans (rotations) n, the slice thickness N·T and the CTDI.

Estimation of effective dose by CTDI

In addition to the comparison of performance against reference dose values, there is sometimes a need to estimate organ doses and the ***effective dose, E*** (ICRP, 1991) for CT procedures to allow risk assessment and comparison with other types of radiological examination. The effective dose for a particular scanning protocol can be estimated from a measured $CTDI_{air}$ value, utilising scanner-specific normalised organ dose data determined for a mathematical anthropomorphic phantom using Monte Carlo techniques (Jones and Shrimpton, 1993; Zankl, 1991).

Alternatively, broad estimates of effective dose can be derived from values of DLP for an examination using appropriately normalised coefficients (EC, 1999):

$$E = E_{DLP} \cdot DLP,$$

where E_{DLP} is the conversion coefficient from dose length product to effective dose, specific to the anatomic region under investigation. The effective dose calculated from DLP values compared with the effective dose based on The NRBP method (Jones et al. 1993) is 15 % lower for the routine chest (Olerud et al. 2001).

Doses in CT of the chest

Table 4.1 gives an analysis of estimated doses calculated for routine chest examinations and HRCT. Imaging and operational parameters have been chosen according to clinical needs (Olerud et al, 2001). The influence of changes in some key technical and operational parameters on the doses is summarised. Such dose data are broadly comparable with practice reported in other countries. Doses from scan projection radiography, also called scout or tomogram image, which is commonly taken to aid localisation in CT scanning, are not included. They contribute only a few percent of total patient dose.

Table 4.1. An analysis of estimated dose values for routine chest CT and HRCT

Scan parameters	Spiral CT of chest	Serial CT of chest	HRCT of chest
Tube voltage (kV)	140	140	140
Tube current (mA)	206	206	111
Rotation time (s)	0,75	0,75	1,5
Current time product/360° (mAs)	154,5	154,5	166,5
Slice thickness (mm)	8	8	1
Table feed/360° (mm)	12	8	10
Number of slices	23	20	22
$CTDI_w$(mGy)	21	21	35
MSAD (mGy)	14	21	3,5
DLP (mGy·cm)	386	336	77
Effective dose (mSv)	6,5	5,6	1,3

While maintaining the imaging parameters (tube voltage, current time product/rotation) nearly constant, the values of MSAD, DLP and effective dose in HRCT with 1 mm slices and 10 mm intervals are about 75 - 80 % lower than in the serial or spiral scanning with conventional 8 mm slices. The $CTDI_w$ is highest in HRCT; the $CTDI_w$ values cannot be used as a criterion for patient exposure, because the dose from 8 mm slices is, in practice, about five times higher than that from 1 mm slices.

Measurement of organ or tissue dose and calculation of effective dose

The effective dose, E, could be calculated from the measurement results of organ or tissue doses with the following expression in publication of ICRP,

$$E=\Sigma w_T H_T ,$$

where w_T is the tissue-weighting factor that represents the relative contribution of the organ or tissue, T, to the total damage caused by irradiation and H_T is the equivalent dose of an organ or tissue, T. The values, w_T, are tabulated in Table 4.2.

The effective dose was primarily defined on the basis of the occupational exposure. To apply the concept of effective dose to the assessment of medical exposure, there are some problems. The occupational exposure is based on the healthy adults ranging from 18 to 65 years old, however those undergone medical exposure range from infants to aged people and are supposed not to be healthy. Additionally, the occupational exposure is assumed to be uniform but the medical exposure is divisional. Since there is no other measure to assess medical exposure, we have to apply the concept of the occupational exposure to the assessment of the medical exposure, with which we can evaluate the medical devices and their examination. The effective dose was used to evaluate the risk described later.

Usually dose measurements are done in the organs or tissues whose tissue weighting factors (W_T) are listed in the 1990 Recommendation of the International Commission on Radiological Protection (ICRP 60, 1990). To measure the dose, the small size detectors are placed in an anthropomorphic tissue equivalent phantom, exposed to the radiation field and then are measured. For this purpose, thermo-luminescent dosimeter (TLD) or the photoluminescence (PL) glass-dosimeter system are appropriate for this purpose. TLD is of cylindrical shape, 2 mm or less in diameter and 10 mm or less in length and the PL glass chip is also of cylindrical shape, 1.5 mm or less in diameter and 12 mm or less in length. There are a variety of detectors of a variety of physical characteristics such as effective atomic number, energy dependency and sensitivity. Generally, energy dependency and sensitivity are complementary and therefore it is important to select suitable detectors according to the purpose.

Table 4.2. Tissue weighting factors (ICRP 60)

Tissue or organ	Tissue weighting factor, W_T
Gonads	0.20
Bone marrow (red)	0.12
Colon	0.12
Lung	0.12
Stomach	0.12
Bladder	0.05
Breast	0.05
Liver	0.05
Oesophagus	0.05
Thyroid	0.05
Skin	0.01
Bone surface	0.01
Remainder*	0.05

For purpose of calculation, the remainder is composed of the following additional tissue and organs: adrenals, brain, small intestine, kidney, muscle, pancreas, spleen, thymus and uterus. The list includes organ which are likely to be selectively irradiated. Some organs in the list are known to be susceptible to cancer induction. If other tissues are having a significant risk of induced cancer they additional list constituting the remainder. The later may also include other tissues or organs selectively irradiated.

Organ or tissue dose evaluation and estimation of effective dose

Nishizawa et al (1995) reported the organ or tissue doses and effective dose in routine chest CT examination with four types of CT. The effective doses were evaluated by the measurement method described in ICRP 60 with an anthropomorphic phantom as mentioned before. Each model was operated in conventional CT scan mode and spiral CT scan mode. The average scan parameters and effective dose of them are listed in Table 4.3.

Table 4.3. Averaged scan parameters and effective dose in routine chest examination

Scan parameter	Conventional CT	Spiral CT
Tube voltage (kV)	120	120
Tube current (mA)	190	165
Scan time (s/rot)	1.125	1.125
Slice thickness / interval (mm)	10/10	10/10
Number of slice	27	27
Effective dose (mSv)	9.2	7.6

Authors measured the organ or tissue doses of the patient during the HRCT examination with an anthropomorphic phantom (Kyoto-Kagaku Inc. Japan, 163cm stature and 53kg weight for whole body) under the current CT examination condition in Japan and that of Nikko Agreement (Chapter 3, Table 3.1) by 2 types of CT apparatus, which are designated as A and B in Table 4.4. The phantom was used as a model of Japanese adult, but the phantom size seems to be smaller than average body size of European or American people. Then the evaluation of organ doses and risk through this phantom measurement is likely to be overestimated for European or American people. Nevertheless, it will be able to show the range of doses and risks.

Table 4.4. Scan parameters and estimated dose values for chest HRCT

	Current condition		Nikko Agreement		
Apparatus	A	B	A[1]	B[1,2]	B[2]
Scan parameter					
Tube voltage (kV)	120	120	120	120	140
Tube current (mA)	200	240	200	200	200
Scan time (s/rot)	1	1	1	1	1
Slice thickness (mm)	2	2	2	2	2
Number of slice	36	11	6	6	6
Organ or tissue doses (mGy)					
Gonad (male)	0.02	0.004	0.01	0.002	0.004
Red bone marrow	4.36	1.20	1.12	0.49	0.70
Lung	13.52	29.5	4.40	1.38	3.22
Thyroid	5.59	1.20	0.92	0.54	0.59
Effective dose (mSv)	5.74	1.69	1.38	0.57	0.93

It can be seen from Table 4.4 that the dose under Nikko Agreement scan condition can be drastically decreased mainly due to the decrease of number of slices. Note also that the dose depends on the device models as seen by the comparison between type A and B. Even with the Nikko Agreement condition, the dose with the Device A is about 2.5 times higher than that of B as seen by the columns A and B superscripted by 1 in Table 4.4. If the tube voltage to a device is varied, the patient dose varies as seen in Columns B superscripted by 2 in Table 4.4. The data with the device B with the tube voltage of 140 kV is intended to show the dose for people of larger body built.

Even though the health examination is done by less exposure than the sequential scanning of all pulmonary area, it is comparatively high according to the current hospital condition. By the condition of Nikko Agreement, the exposure dose can be greatly decreased.

Risk evaluation

Epidemiological studies of irradiated populations

Numerous studies have demonstrated increased risks of cancer and other health effects due to radiation exposure among various populations. These populations include patients who were irradiated for diagnostic or therapeutic reasons (UNSCEAR 2000) as well as radiation workers in nuclear industry (Cardis *et al* 1995, Muirhead *et al* 1999, Iwasaki *et al* 2003) and medical profession (Yoshinaga *et al*), and atomic bomb survivors in Japan (Thompson *et al* 1994, Preston *et al* 1994, Pierce *et al* 1996, Shimizu *et al* 1999). Epidemiological studies of atomic bomb survivors is the main source to provide direct evidence of radiation-induced cancer that is considered as the most important health effect due to radiation exposure. However, atomic bomb survivors received single exposure to moderate-to-high dose of radiation at high dose rate. The cancer risk of low dose of radiation, e.g., under 200 mSv, has not been well clarified by epidemiological studies or animal studies.

Assessment of cancer risk due to HRCT exposure

As described in the previous chapter, the magnitude of exposure doses from HRCT was estimated, at most, to be 4.5 mGy for organ or tissue dose and 1.4 mSv for whole body effective dose under the condition of the Nikko Agreement. According to UNSCEAR 2000 report, worldwide average annual dose from natural radiation is 2.4 mSv, comprising 0.39 mSv from cosmic X-ray, 0.48 mSv from terrestrial external radiation, 1.26 from radon and its decay products, and 0.29 mSv from internal exposure from foodstuff. It should be noted that there is a large variation in dose from natural radiation between nations or individuals. An expected increase of risk due to HRCT exposure would be small at such low doses with low statistical power to detect the increased risk. In addition, other factors than HRCT exposure would confound the effect of interest. In such situation, the HRCT-related risk cannot be easily discriminated from that of other sources of radiation even in a well-designed epidemiological study. Extrapolation of risks from high dose to low dose is commonly used to assess cancer risks at low dose, which is often referred as "risk projection". Risk projection can be a useful alternative of epidemiological studies to get a quantitative estimate of the risk due to HRCT exposures.

Measures of radiation risk due to HRCT exposure

In the risk projection, several measures can be used to quantify risks (UNSCEAR 1994). First, "loss of life expectancy (LLE)" is the difference of the expectation of life between individuals with and without exposure to radiation, e.g., HRCT. LLE for an individual exposed to dose D at age e is given by

$$LLE(D,e) = \int_e^\infty S(a|e)da - \int_e^\infty S(a|D,e)da$$

where S(a|D,e) and S(a|e) indicate the probability that an individual with and without exposure to dose D at age e, survives to age a given that he or she was alive at age e.

Another measure of the risk is "excess lifetime risk (ELR)". The definition of the ELR is the difference of the proportions of people dying of cancer in their life among a target population (e.g., with HRCT exposure) and among a similar population (e.g., without HRCT exposure). ELR for an individual exposed to dose D at age e is given by

$$ELR(D,e) = \int_e^\infty m(a|D,e)S(a|D,e)da - \int_e^\infty m(a)S(a|e)da$$

where m(a|D,e) and m(a) indicate the mortality rates from cause of interest at age a with and without exposure to dose D at age e, and other quantities are the same as in the definition of LLE.

"Risk of exposure-induced death (REID)" is also used as a measure of radiation risk. This is a probability that an individual would die of a cancer that occurred, in his/her life, due to the exposure of interest. REID for an individual exposed to dose D at age e is given by

$$REID(D,e) = \int_e^\infty [m(a|D,e) - m(a)]S(a|D,e)da$$

where quantities are the same as in the definition of LLE or ELR.

These three measures describe the impact of exposure on an exposed population regardless of whether an event actually occurred in an individual in the population. On the other hand, if the LLE is divided by the REID, this measure becomes years of life lost per radiation-induced case (YLC), describing the impact of exposure on an individual whose cause of death is radiation exposure of interest.

Above measures of risk are derived from life-table method for which basic data are needed on age- and sex-specific distribution of target population, corresponding background mortality, and risk models with risk coefficients. The two types of risk models are commonly used for the risk projection, i.e., absolute risk model under which excess mortality depends on a risk coefficient that is often expressed as excess absolute risk (EAR), and exposure dose, and relative risk model under which excess cancer mortality depends on background mortality rates as well as on a risk coefficient that is often expressed as excess relative risk (ERR), and exposure dose.

Estimates of radiation risk due to HRCT exposure

The four measures of risk from HRCT exposure were calculated. All cancers except leukemia and lung cancer, were considered in the calculation because other sites of cancer have lower radiation sensitivity or lower background mortality. Table 4.5 shows the assumptions for the risk calculation. For the calculation of risks of all cancers except leukemia and lung cancer, we assumed a 10-year latent period and a constant ERR after the period. For leukemia risk calculation, we assumed a 2-year latent period and a constant EAR until 40 year after exposure, with zero risk after then. In the calculation, the life-table and cause-age-specific cancer mortality of Japanese population in 2000 was used. The risk coefficients, i.e., ERR or EAR per Sv/Gy were derived from mortality data for atomic bomb survivors between 1950 and 1990 (Pierce et al 1996). Although data on atomic bomb survivors indicate ERR and EAR depend on age at exposure and/or time since exposure (Pierce et al, 1996), our calculation was based on simple assumption with no time dependency. A reduction factor is widely used for the effect of low dose and/or low dose-rate of exposure, but this factor was not taken into account here.

Table 4.5. Assumptions for lifetime risk calculation

Cancer sites	Dose for calculation	Risk model	Risk coefficient	Latent period	Projection methods
All except for leukemia	1.38 mSv (effective dose)	Relative risk model	0.38 per Sv (ERR)	10 years	ERR is assumed constant from 10 years after exposure
Lung	4.40 mGy (lung dose)	Relative risk model	0.30 per Sv (ERR)	10 years	ERR is assumed constant from 10 years after exposure
Leukemia	1.12 mGy (red bone marrow dose)	Absolute risk model	3.45 per 10^4 person-year·Sv (EAR)	2 years	EAR is assumed constant from 2 years and zero from 40 years after exposure

Note: ERR, excess relative risk. EAR, excess absolute risk. ATE, age at exposure

Table 4.6 shows ELR, REID, LLE, and YLC for all cancers except leukemia, lung cancer, and leukemia due to HRCT exposure under the condition of Nikko Agreement (Chapter 3, Table 3.1). Risks from such low dose exposure from HRCT are very small regardless of measures of risk. It should be mentioned that these estimates of the risks would vary according to different assumption on risk models, projection methods, background mortality, etc.

Table 4.6. Estimated risks of selected cancers due to HRCT exposure (Nikko Agreement, Table 3.1, Chapter 3)

Age at exposure	Type of cancer	ELR (%)	REID (%)	LLE (years)	YLC (years)
30	All except leukemia	0.0122	0.0157	0.0018	12
	Lung	0.0086	0.0091	0.0010	11
	Leukemia	0.0014	0.0014	0.0004	29
50	All except leukemia	0.0115	0.0148	0.0015	10
	Lung	0.0083	0.0088	0.0009	10
	Leukemia	0.0007	0.0007	0.0001	20

Risk-benefit analysis is of value to examine the usefulness of HRCT or other medical procedures. Nishizawa *et al* performed a risk-benefit analysis for lung cancer screening CT, showing that the benefit will exceed the risk for Japanese over forty years of age for men and over forty-five for women. However, the benefit of HRCT use, such as decrease of mortality or prolongation of life after finding early stage of lung disease cannot be easily quantified without various assumptions. A controlled trial can provide direct evidence of the benefit and risk of HRCT screening, although it has not become available to date. Judging from current scientific knowledge of the effects of exposure to low dose radiation, the risk from HRCT screening would be negligible, and its use can be justified.

Reference

ICRP (1996). Radiological protection and safety in medicine. ICRP Publication 73. Annals of the ICRP 26(2). Pergamon Press, Oxford

European Commission (1999). Quality Criteria for Computed Tomography, European Guidelines (1999). CEC document, EUR 16262, Luxembourg

DHHS, FDA (1984) CFR Part 1020: Diagnostic X-ray Systems and Their Major Components; Amendments to Performance Standard; Final Rule. Federal Register, 49: 171

IEC, International Electrotechnical Commission (2001). Medical Electrical Equipment - Part 2. Particular requirements for the safety of x-ray equipment for computed tomography. IEC Standard 60601-2-44, edn 2,. IEC, Geneva

IEC, Amendment 1 to IEC 60601-2-44 (2001). Medical Electrical Equipment, Part 2-44: Particular Requirements for the Safety of X-ray Equipment for Computed tomography, Iec,Geneva

ICRP (1991). 1990 Recommendations of the International Commission on Radiological Protection. ICRP Publication 60. Annals of the ICRP 21 Nos 1-3, Pergamon Press, Oxford

Jones, D.G. and P.C. Shrimpton (1993). Normalised organ doses for x-ray computed tomography calculated using Monte Carlo techniques. NRPB-SR250. NRPB, Chilton

Zankl, M.,W. Panzer and G. Drexler (1991). The calculation of dose from external photon exposures using reference human phantoms and Monte Carlo methods. Part VI: Organ doses from computed tomographic examinations. GSF-Berich 30/91. GSF, Neuherberg

Olerud HM, Torp CG, Einarsson G, Grön P, Leitz W, Servomaa A. Use of the EC quality criteria as a common method of inspecting CT laboratories- a pilot project by the Nordic radiation protection authorities. Proc. Int. Conf

Radiological Protection of Patients in Diagnostic and Interventional Radiology. Malaga. Marc 26-30.2001. IAEA, Vienna

Shope TB, Gagne RM, Johnson GC (1981) A method for describing the doses delivered by transmission x-ray computed tomography. Med Phys. 8:488-495

Itoh S, Ikeda M, Arahata S et al. (2000). Lung cancer screening: minimum tube current required for helical CT. Radiology 215 (1): 175-183

UNSCEAR (2000) United Nations Scientific Committee on the Effects of Atomic Radiation. 2000 Report to the General Assembly, Annex D: Medical Radiation Exposures. United Nations, New York NY

van der Bruggen-Bogaarts BA, Broerse JJ, Lammers JW, van Waes PF, Geleijns J. Radiation exposure in standard and high-resolution chest CT scans. Chest 107; 113-5, 1995

Nishizawa K, Maruyama T, Takayama M, Iwai K, Furuya Y: Estimetion of effective dose from CT examination. Nippon Acta Radiologica 55; 763-768,1995

Yoshinaga S, Mabuchi K, Sigurdson AJ, Doody MM, Ron E. Cancer risks among radiologists and radiologic technologists: A review of epidemiological studies, submitted

Nishizawa K, Iwai K, Matsumoto T, Sakashita K, Iinuma A, Tateno Y, Miyamoto T. Estimation of the exposure and a risk-benefit analysis for a CT system designed for a lung cancer mass screening unit. Radiat Prot Dosim 1996; 67:101-108

Ministry of Health and Welfare, Japan. The 19th life tables. Health and welfare statistics association. Tokyo, 2002 (ISSN 0911-8500)

Cardis E, Gilbert ES, Carpenter L, Howe G, Kato I, Armstrong BK, Beral V, Cowper G, Douglas G, Wiggs LD. Effects of low doses and low dose rates of external ionizing radiation: cancer mortality among nuclear workers in three countries. Radiat Res 1995; 142:117-132

Muirhead CR, Goodill AA, Haylock RGE, Vokes J, Little MP, Jackson DA, O'Hagan JA, Thomas JM, Kendall GM, Berridge GLC. Occupational radiation exposure and mortality: Second analysis of the National Registry of Radiation Workers. J Radiol Prot 1999; 19:3-26

Iwasaki T, Murata M, Ohshima S, Miyake T, Kudo S, Inoue Y, Narita M, Yoshimura T, Akiba S, Tango T, Yoshimoto Y, Shimizu Y, Sobue T, Kusumi S, Yamagishi C, Matsudaira H. Second analysis of mortality of nuclear industry workers in Japan, 1986-1997. Radiat Res 2003; 159:228-238

Pierce DA, Shimizu Y, Preston DL, Vaeth M, Mabuchi K. Studies of the mortality of atomic bomb survivors. Report 12, Part 1. Cancer: 1950-1990. Radiat Res 1996; 146:1-27

Shimizu Y, Pierce DA, Preston DL, Mabuchi K. Studies of the mortality of atomic bomb survivors. Report 12, Part 1. Non-cancer mortality: 1950-1990. Radiat Res 1999; 152:374-389

Thompson DE, Mabuchi K, Ron E, Soda M, Tokunaga M, Ochikubo S, Sugimoto S, Ikeda T, Terasaki M, Izumi S. Cancer incidence in atomic bomb survivors. Part II: Solid tumors: 1958-1987. Radiat Res 1994; 137: S17-S67

Preston DL, Kusumi S, Tomonaga M, Izumi S, Ron E, Kuramoto A, Kamada N, Dohy H, Matsuo T. Cancer incidence in atomic bomb survivors. Part III. Leukemia, lymphoma, and multiple myeloma: 1950-1987. Radiat Res 1994; 137:S68-S97

UNSCEAR 1994. Sources and effects of ionizing radiation, Annex A. Epidemiological studies of radiation carcinogenesis. United Nations, New York. 1994

Chapter 5 Application of the International Classification of HRCT for the Occupational Lung Diseases

Narufumi Suganuma and Yukinori Kusaka

Department of Environmental Health, School of Medicine, Fukui Medical University, 23-3 Shimoaizuki, Matsuoka, Yoshida, Fukui 910-1193, Japan

Introduction

Applying computed tomography (CT) to the occupational lung diseases has been an attempt to understand morphological feature of respiratory manifestation more adjacent to pathology. It has been introduced as a thorough investigation for positive cases screened by chest radiograph. The high-resolution CT (HRCT) provides higher spatial resolution to enable us to recognise morphologic changes of secondary lobule (Itoh et al. 1978). When it is introduced into screening for early detection of occupational lung diseases, it will shift the scheme of screening for dust-induced respiratory diseases from detection of definite cases to recognition of the earliest manifestation of the diseases (Fig. 5.1).

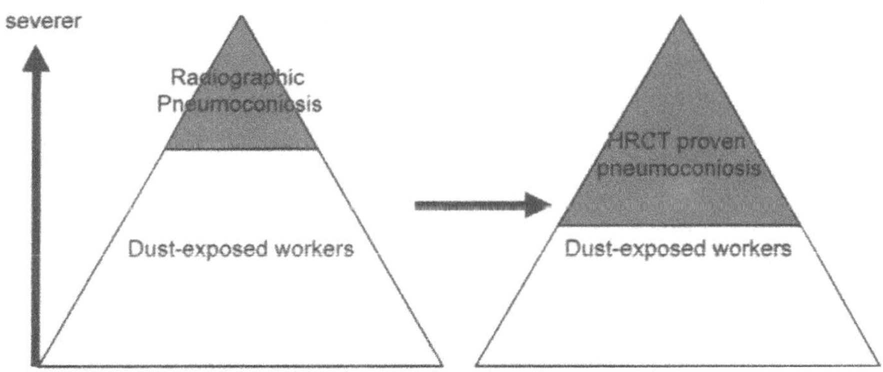

Fig.5.1. Introducing HRCT into screening for pneumoconioses enables an earliest preventive intervention to dust exposed workers. Note severity of pneumoconiosis progresses upward usually as latent period and amount of dust-exposure increases

The purpose of the ILO 2000 International Classification of Radiograph for Pneumoconioses (ILO 2000) is to classify dust-exposed workers with moderate chest roentgenogram (CXR) manifestation and to make intervention to stop them from further exposure to dust. This ILO system is well organised and has minor disagreement among trained readers, especially when classifying the profusion of small opacities. However, as pneumoconioses are progressive diseases without curative therapy, it seems to be too late to detect moderate cases for intervention. Also a well-spread awareness of asbestos a as definite carcinogen among workers has lead to demand more sensitive screening for asbestos-related respiratory diseases.

It is well recognised that HRCT gives clear view both for parenchymal and pleural abnormalities. However, standard textbooks on the occupational lung disease often deny possibility of using HRCT for screening purposes (Bretland 1994). Cost and availability of the test as well as radiation dose with usual scan will be the reasons why HRCT are excluded from screening tests (Table 5.1). In order to overcome these shortcomings, low dose technique is introduced into HRCT, in which dose with as low as plain chest radiograph can be obtained. Also for the purpose of screening, limited number of slices is reported to be enough for detecting occupational lung diseases, especially asbestosis (Aberle et al. 1988; Friedman et al. 1988; Gamsu et al. 1989; Staples 1992). For detailed discussion on dose reduction effect by introducing the Nikko Agreement, see Chapter 4 (Table 4.6) by Nishizawa et al., this volume.

Table 5.1. Application of radiological diagnostic tests for screening, surveillance and clinical diagnosis

Diagnostic test	Radiation dose (mSv)	Time for exam (min)	Data	Cost per test	Screening	Surveillance	Clinical Diagnosis
CXR	0.05	within 5	film	$20	good	good	minimum
DR	0.05	within 5	digital	$20	good	good	minimum
helical CT	1.0* - 9.5	20	digital	$100	for cancer, conditional	for cancer, conditional	good
HRCT	1.0* - 9.5	20	digital	$100	for OERD, conditional	for OERD, condtional	good
MDCT	1.0* - 9.5	20	digital	$100	for both	for both	good

Note that abbreviations are as follows. CXR: chest radiograph; DR: digital chest radiograph; CT: computed tomography; HRCT: high-resolution or thin slice CT; MDCT: multi-detector CT and OERD: occupational and environmental respiratory diseases.
*When low dose protocol (Nikko Agreement, Table 3.1, Chapter 3) is applied.

Rather experimental screening programmes performed in Germany (Kraus et al. 1996), France and Finland (Huuskonen et al. 2001) are among those targeted both for benign and malignant asbestos-induced respiratory diseases. Their programme use combination of selected slices of HRCT and a whole lung spiral CT.

There are many questions to be asked when introducing this International Classification of HRCT for the Occupational and Environmental Respiratory Diseases into screening programme for population at risk of developing the occupational lung diseases. How could the Classification be used in various setting? Is it for the purpose of academic research? Is it for radiologists, or for pulmonary physicians? Or is it practical enough to be used in clinic to assess dust-exposed individuals? Are the readings by different readers standardised enough to give grades of pneumoconiotic findings? Could the positive findings by the Classification automatically be interpreted as pneumoconioses? How can we accumulate the data and utilise them for prevention of dust-induced pulmonary diseases? We will try to answer these questions.

Application of the Classification may differ from country to country in which the Classification is applied as measure of secondary prevention of dust-induced respiratory diseases. It may depend on availability of the CT apparatus, implication of CT screening for dust-exposed individuals, social interest or needs for dust-induced respiratory diseases, and so forth. In fact, although 67% of Japanese hospitals possessed CT scanner, and even though this percentage is exceptionally high, CT screening is not obligatory for pneumoconioses according to governmental regulations. Japan has been using chest X-ray for legitimate screening of dust-exposed workers since 1960. Recently, the Scientific Committee of Ministry of Health, Welfare and Labour, Japan has recommended pneumoconiotics to undertake annual spiral CT exam in order to screen for lung cancer and the Pneumoconioses Law has been revised to include the statement.

On the other hand, some European countries, namely Finland (Huuskonen et al. 2001), Germany (Kraus et al. 1996) and France (De Vuyst 2000) have started HRCT screening programme. These countries are economically matured enough but the CT scanner is not as abundant as Japan. In these countries, a need for screening for lung cancer and mesothelioma among asbestos-exposed workers has arisen, because it is socially recognised that asbestos is a carcinogenic dust. Helsinki criteria (Anonymous 1997) agreed in 1997 may have convinced European researchers to introduce HRCT for screening for earlier manifestation of asbestosis or asbestos-related pleural abnormalities than irregular opacity 1/0 of radiograph by ILO 1980. By the utilisation of the HRCT Classification, earlier recognition of dust-induced the occupational lung diseases would become possible and the positive-test individuals will increase largely in number, and when the causative dust is carcinogenic they are subjected to cancer screening by spiral CT.

As described above, target diseases of medical screenings for dust-exposed individuals are of two kinds, one is for detection of non-malignant respiratory diseases and the other is for that of malignant diseases. Although screening of dust-exposed individuals for medical assessment for pneumoconioses has been performed in most of developed countries, not many countries have introduced screening programme for occupational lung cancer. Japanese Pneumoconiosis

Law legitimates medical screening by chest X-ray for dust-exposed workers against dust-induced benign respiratory diseases, and for individuals with carcinogenic dust exposure another law legitimates chest X-ray for detection of malignant respiratory diseases. German researchers have already developed CT/HRCT classification to detect very subtle findings up to tumours and have performed survey over 600 dust-exposed workers (Woitowitz and Kraus 2000). In their protocol non-malignant respiratory diseases were screened by HRCT, while malignant respiratory diseases were screened by spiral CT. The latter technique has low resolution than HRCT but, theoretically, has no gap between slices. Similar practice was made by Finnish group (Huuskonen et al. 2001). They have developed their own Fibrosis Grading system to assess clinical severity of each case by HRCT. Their results showed the superiority of the grading by HRCT to ILO 1980 Classification through receiver operating curve (ROC) analysis (Fig. 5.2).

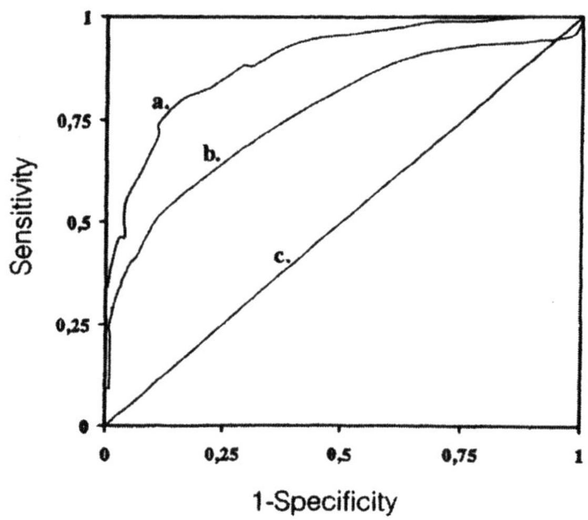

Fig. 5.2. Curves of the receiver operating characteristic (ROC) classification. [a = high-resolution computed tomography (HRCT) fibrosis score, b = classification of the International Labour Office (ILO), c = 0.5 reference line] (from Huuskonenn et al. 2001, with permission)

The purpose of the HRCT Classification is to describe and code parenchymal and pleural manifestation of diffuse non-malignant occupational and environmental respiratory diseases. The Classification gives a semi-quantitative tool for early detection of fibrotic changes induced by occupational and environmental dust-exposure. Positive scoring by the HRCT Classification does not always mean the presence of pneumoconioses. Therefore, it could be used in following three settings.

Clinical Diagnosis

The Classification system is not originally designated for clinical diagnosis of the occupational lung diseases. Usually, in clinical setting, most of HRCT films will be assessed by pulmonary radiologists in well-equipped general hospitals, because such hospitals can afford to be equipped with the CT scanners. The patient will be referred to those hospitals and HRCT will be subsequent examination to chest-X-ray with positive findings. Low dose HRCT will not be applicable in this setting.

However, the Classification could be used in clinical setting with modification. The reading sheet of the classification (Fig. 2.1, Chapter 2) gives physician a checklist of possible manifestation of the occupational lung diseases when reviewing HRCT of patients with or without dust-exposure. The reference film set in accompany (CD-ROM) is also useful to know typical parenchymal and pleural manifestation of dust-induced respiratory diseases. A set of the Classification, included in this handy book, can be utilised in educating residents or physicians who are not familiar with pneumoconioses. This system will be soon prepared as a computer-assisted system (Kraus et al. 1997). Clinicians, in near future, may look at patient's HRCT scan and the reference slice of the Classification side-by-side on the monitor.

Another benefit of introducing the Classification into clinical works is that we have standard scale to evaluate HRCT of the dust-exposed. One radiologist may diagnoses HRCT with grade 1 intralobular irregular opacities as 'definite pulmonary fibrosis', while other may call it 'mild fibrotic changes'. Several studies performed by authors have described possible variation of HRCT reading results even among experts of occupational lung diseases (Suganuma et al. 2001). This strongly suggests definite need for standardising readers' quality when using the Classification into practical use. Using grade referring to the same reference films set, we can share what we saw in more quantitative and comparative way. This will accelerate our accumulation of knowledge on the HRCT findings of the diseases.

Evidence-based medicine requires physicians to have their own practice to be related to epidemiologic knowledge. Accumulation of clinical data in standardised way using the HRCT Classification system will help to perform clinical epidemiologic studies.

Screening

Purpose of medical screening is to detect disease in its pre-clinical stage to benefit an individual underwent a certain diagnostic test. When we look at two populations either with or without a disease, *e.g.* pneumoconiosis, the meaning of screening becomes much easier to understand. Any diagnostic test does not accurately decide whether a person has disease or not. Most of the positive-test individuals have disease and most of the negative-test individuals do not have disease, but there are some who are test positive and do not have disease and others who are test negative but with disease. According to the ILO 1980 Classification of Radiograph, the profusion 1/0 is, by definition, considered to be positive and 0/1 is negative. The distinction between 0/1 and 1/0 is called cut-off point of the screening test, *i.e.* chest X-ray, for pneumoconiosis. Cut-off point of the screening test is decided as suited for the purpose of the test, basically maximising sensitivity and/or specificity of the test. Sensitive test will detect most of the disease, while specific test will detect most of the disease free individuals. When sensitivity changes from 1 to 0, specificity moves from 0 to 1. Thus, there is trade-off between sensitivity and specificity and we cannot have them both 1, lest we use the very same test as a golden standard, which means that there is always false positive and false negative cases. The trade-off between sensitivity and specificity is well described by receiver operating curve (ROC) (see Fig. 5.2). When the purpose of the screening test is to detect malignant disease, increasing sensitivity of the test is more important than increasing specificity. On the other hand, high specific screening test will be appropriate for detecting benign diseases.

Another aspect of screening test is positive predictive value that shows ratio of true positive cases among test positive individuals. Number of false positive and false negative cases differs when populations differs, because it depends on the prevalence of target disease for which the screening test is applied. In practice, this positive predictive value decides number of test-positive individuals among the tested people when the prevalence of the disease in the population is given. Thus, the process of selecting a population to apply a screening programme is the very important part in the assessment whether a proposed programme is cost-effective or not.

Application of screening programme should be carefully assessed by following conditions that Wagner (Wagner 1996) summarised. He states that the disease "*(1) causes significant morbidity and mortality; (2) can be identified at a pre-symptomatic stage before the individual would ordinarily seek medical care; (3) responds to acceptable, available and effective intervention and treatment; (4) is prevalent in the population undergoing screening.*" And that the test "*(1) is acceptable to those at risk for disease; (2) has adequate sensitivity, specificity and predictive value in the target population; (3) is available at a reasonable cost; (4) is sufficiently standardised to be performed with consistency, accuracy and reproducibility.*"

The disease targeted by the HRCT Classification is the occupational lung diseases whose prevalence among dust-exposed workers is high enough as 15.1% (2857/18,900) (Koskinen et al. 1998). As HRCT will detect pulmonary involvement of the occupational lung diseases earlier than conventional radiographs, intervention to exposed individuals in earlier stages than 1/0 of ILO1980 would show better response. As stated in Chapter 3, low dose scan will produce sufficient image for screening purpose. Cost of the screening HRCT scan plus spiral CT is about 20 times as radiograph, and whether this is cost effective or not is subjected to further study. However, as thin- and thick slice section had become able to be obtained by single multi-detector CT (MDCT) scan, MDCT may become standard tool for the occupational lung diseases screening. At least we have just cleared the last condition listed above (4), the standardisation of screening protocol (Anonymous 2000).

Surveillance

Surveillance is a public health practice for disease prevention by continuing collection of health-related data, analysing them and distributing the results to applicable person. It is more emphasised to obtain health related information of population in surveillance rather than early detection of a disease for an individual as in medical screening (CDC 1988). Data utilised for surveillance could be any accumulated data, including environmental monitoring or social statistics as well as individual laboratory data. Any health statistics accumulated at health department of national government, or environmental chemical substances monitored by strategic sampling system can be subjected to surveillance. In workplaces environmental hazard is monitored and at the same time adverse health effect of the hazard on workers is also monitored periodically.

As for pneumoconioses, radiographic change as well as environmental dust concentration is monitored in dusty workplaces. The surveillance could utilise individual clinical data obtained at hospital or private medical doctors when its purpose is to monitor health problem among population at risk of the occupational lung diseases. The definition of the disease or health problems to be surveyed or monitored, of course, should be clearly stated and same standardised method should be used.

When the Classification system is introduced widely into many hospitals and clinics, number of data on dust-exposed individuals screened by HRCT will be accumulated. We furthermore have to analyse and distribute the data to healthcare staffs, workplaces and workers continuously in order to establish surveillance system. The target diseases of the Classification system, however, do not require as quick response as the surveillance against communicable diseases, as the former diseases usually progress with more continuous exposure and longer latent periods than the latter do. Anyhow, as surveillance system needs real time reporting and quick response to the possible clustering of target diseases, computerisation of the Classification system will accelerate to develop such network.

Linkage of screening data and referral hospital data would be expected when assessing the screening programme, and following up dust-exposed populations. The data accumulated by the screening programme and those by referral hospitals should be separately analysed because prevalence of the occupational lung diseases among population underwent HRCT examination will differ widely. Information technology is well developed enough to provide secure and speedy communication system for the purpose.

Expected effect of the surveillance using HRCT is knowledge on prevalence of the occupational lung diseases among dust-exposed individuals or in general population, which reflect dose of dust-exposure among the population. As some of the dust has been shown to be carcinogenic, surveillance for malignant diseases should be jointly performed. Workers using newly synthesised and hazardous, sometimes carcinogenic, substances in dust form should also be surveyed with this sensitive method for possible respiratory adverse effect.

Table 5.1 summarised bilateral aspects of several radiological diagnostic tests possibly used for screening, surveillance or clinical diagnosis of the occupational lung diseases. The line to divide appropriate screening measure for the occupational lung diseases will be drawn with considerable variation in social situation among countries. Introduction of low dose CT and HRCT will allow the Classification system to be used for screening and surveillance. The technique itself is of course for diagnosis of the occupational lung diseases and, as described previously, the system may give valuable checklist and sample slices for clinicians when interpreting HRCT findings of dust-exposed individuals.

When the impact of the disease to individuals is considered, cancer screening will prevail to benign the occupational lung diseases screening. There have been reports from Japan (Sone et al. 1998) and from USA (Henschke et al. 2001) on similar spiral CT screening for lung cancer. These successful reports have encouraged us to perform similar screening programme among population at higher risk of occupational lung cancer and mesothelioma than usual tobacco smoking subjects. However, last expert meeting did not declared introduction of this new screening method for cancer detection among dust-exposed population. This seemed to be rather conservative but the consensus report recognises potential efficacy of new methods. When spiral CT screening for cancer and mesothelioma is justified, HRCT is then needed to define population at higher risk to be subjected to cancer screening (Fig. 5.3).

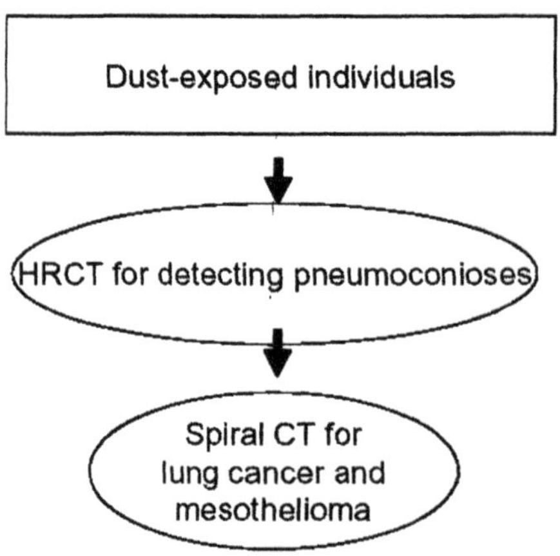

Fig. 5.3. Screening of workers exposed to carcinogenic dust like asbestos. HRCT is a tool for detecting benign respiratory diseases, and spiral CT a lung cancer detector

Reliability and Education

Reliability of the screening and surveillance consist of various factors that build up its system, but one of the most important factor is repeatability of reading results among the physicians who read the CT films and use the Classification. Our study revealed satisfactory repeatability among multinational physicians with considerable experience in management of pneumoconiotic patients (Suganuma et al, submitted). This result should be tested among physicians with various backgrounds and also with less experience in this field.

As the purpose of the Classification is standardization of CT reading among physicians, it needs education tools and system that gives certain standard that the users can rely on. We have held 2 days' workshop for radiologists, pulmonologists, and occupational physicians on radiological images of pneumoconioses in Tsuruga, Japan in November 2000. That was a view-box seminar, in which participants could practice reading CXR and CT films with reference to the ILO or the CT Classifications.

Standardisation is now on-going in various fields. The benefit of this time consuming effort is globalisation of the field, which enables us to share experiences internationally, and to minimise future effort to harmonise similar domestic standards. At least participants of the HRCT project will share their experiences in their field of practice, clinics, workplaces, screening trial field and so forth to deepen their knowledge on epidemiology, radiology, pathology, occupational and environmental medicine of the occupational and environmental respiratory diseases.

The twenty-first century is the era of network. The distribution and popularisation of the CT Classification system will proceed not from orthodox vertical way but from everywhere. As long as the classification is well organised and further application is proposed continuously, the Classification will diffusely distributed spontaneously.

Further accumulation of research on the HRCT Classification is needed to establish world wide surveillance system for the occupational lung diseases. Among the expected work will be pilot screening programme for benign occupational lung diseases by the Classification and assessment of listed findings on the Reading Sheet (Fig. 2.1, Chapter 2) to select most attributable to severity of clinical stage, prognosis or malignant complication of the occupational lung diseases. Mathematical modelling using the selected factors will provide us computerised HRCT diagnosis assistant system for the occupational lung diseases.

Conclusions

As stated above, the Classification is designated for the purpose of medical screening and surveillance for the occupational lung diseases. However, the set of classification included in this book will give assistance also in clinical diagnosis of the occupational lung diseases. Wide application of the Classification is expected for further understanding of prevalence, prognosis and complications of the occupational lung diseases.

References

Anonymous (1997). Asbestos, asbestosis, and cancer: the Helsinki criteria for dignosis and attribution. Scand J Work Environ Health 23: 311-316

Anonymous (2000). International expert meeting on new advances in the radiology and screening of asbestos-related diseases. Scand J Work Environ Health 26(5): 449-454

Aberle, D. R., G. Gamsu, et al. (1988). Asbestos-related pleural and parenchymal fibrosis: detection with high- resolution CT. Radiology 166(3): 729-34

Bretland, P. M. (1994). Imaging in occupational disease of the lung. Part III: Other imageing techniques. Occupational Lung Disorders. W. Raymond Parkes. Oxford, Butterworth Heinemann: 192-196

CDC (1988). Guidelines for evaluating surveillance systems. MMWR 37(S5): 1-18

De Vuyst, P. (2000). Recommendation of the French consensus meeting. An International Expert Meeting on New Advances in Radiology and Screening of Asbestos-Related Diseases, Espoo, Finland, Finnish Institute of Occupational Health

Friedman, A. C., S. B. Fiel, et al. (1988). Asbestos-related pleural disease and asbestosis: a comparison of CT and chest radiography. Am J Roentgenol 150(2): 269-75

Gamsu, G., D. R. Aberle, et al. (1989). Computed tomography in the diagnosis of asbestos-related thoracic disease. J Thorac Imaging 4(1): 61-7

Henschke, C. I., D. P. Naidich, et al. (2001). Early lung cancer action project: initial findings on repeat screenings. Cancer 92(1): 153-9

Huuskonen, O., L. Kivisaari, et al. (2001). High-resolution computed tomography classification of lung fibrosis for patients with asbestos-related disease. Scand J Work Environ Health 27(2): 106-12

Itoh, H., S. Tokunaga, et al. (1978). Radiologic-pathologic correlations of small lung nodules with special reference to peribronchiolar nodules. Am J Roentgenol 130: 223-231

Koskinen, K., A. Zitting, et al. (1998). Radiographic abnormalities among Finnish construction, shipyard and asbestos industry workers. Scand J Work Environ Health 24(2): 109-17

Kraus, T., H. J. Raithel, et al. (1996). Evaluation and classification of high-resolution computed tomographic findings in patients with pneumoconiosis. Int Arch Occup Environ Health 68(4): 249-54

Kraus, T., H. J. Raithel, et al. (1997). Computer-assisted classification system for chest X-ray and computed tomography findings in occupational lung disease. Int Arch Occup Environ Health 69(6): 482-6

Sone, S., S. Takashima, et al. (1998). Mass screening for lung cancer with mobile spiral computed tomography scanner. Lancet 351(9111): 1242-5

Staples, C. A. (1992). Computed tomography in the evaluation of benign asbestos-related disorders. Radiol Clin North Am 30(6): 1191-207

Suganuma, N., Y. Kusaka, et al. (2001). The Japanese Classification of Computed Tomography for Pneumoconioses with Standard Films: Comparison with the ILO International Classification of Radiographs for Pneumoconioses. J Occup Health 43(1): 24-31

Suganuma, N., Y. Kusaka, et al. The development of the Classification of HRCT for Occupational and Environmental Respiratory Diseases. Int Arch Occup Environ Health (submitted)

Wagner, G. R. (1996). Screening and surveillance of workers exposed to mineral dusts. Geneva, World Health Organisation

Woitowitz, H. J. and T. Kraus (2000). Screening of asbestos-exposed workers in Germany. An International Expert Meeting on New Advances in Radiology and Screening of Asbestos-Related Diseases, Espoo, Finland, Finnish Institute of Occupational Health

Chapter 6 ILO International Classifications of Radiographs of Pneumoconioses – Past, Present and Future –

Yutaka Hosoda

Consultant, Radiation Effects Research Foundation, Hijiyama Park 5-2, Minami-ku, Hiroshima, 732-0815, Japan

The ILO International Classification of Pneumoconioses is an internationally used system to identify and record radiographic changes provoked by industrial dusts. The preliminary classification was first proposed at the 1930 International Conference on Silicosis held in Johanesburg South Africa and the prototype of the present classification was made in 1950 for pulmonary abnormalities due to mineral dust exposures. Since then, the scope has been expanded to exposures to all other dusts to keep pace with the industrial changes. This chapter is concerned with the guidelines and standard radiographs of the 1950, 1958, 1968, 1971, 1980 and 2000 versions. A look to the future is also included.

Initial or Pioneering Classifications : Profusion or Size/Type

Before use of radiographs, pneumoconiosis was evaluated by working capacity. When radiographs came to wide use, various radiological classifications were developed in industrial countries such as Britain, France, Germany, South Africa, United States, and former USSR in 1930s and 1940s (1-8), mostly combined with clinical findings, as seen in the recommendation by the 1930 International Conference on Silicosis held in Johannesburg. In radiographical classifications, there were two major schools. One is the classification with emphasis of profusion of discrete small shadows as represented by the Welsh National Memorial Association (1931) and British Medical Research Council Pneumoconiosis Research Unit (PRU, 1945) and the other that stressing the dominant morphological size/type of such shadows as represented by French and Belgian groups (6).

Internationally Agreed Classifications (Tables 6.1 and 6.2)

The 1950 International Labour Office (ILO) Sydney Classification

Scope: Mineral dusts

With some degree of international agreement at the 1950 Sydney Meeting, ILO issued “a suggested international scheme of the classification of radiographs in some of the pneumoconioses” mainly for coalmines, but also for other industries. The size/type of shadow was put outside of the main classification, but allowed to be used if considered important. When small opacities are unevenly distributed in different areas of the lung fields, the profusion category is determined by the most advanced abnormality that is present in at least half of a lung field. This concept differs from the 1980 guidelines mentioning the consideration of profusion in 6 lung zones in both sides. In those days, coalescent opacities were so frequently combined with tuberculosis that separation of the two diseases was difficult (silico-tuberculosis) .

It should be noted that the experts participating in this 1950 conference were wise enough to avoid terms suggesting a definite process of development, or a definite pathogenesis such as “initial”, “terminal”, “progressive”, “infective”, in describing radiographic features. As for the definition of classifications, higher priority was usually put on standard reference films than verbal definitions. As film-to-film copying techniques were not available at that time, each reference film set contained different original radiographs (Personal communications with J Gilson, then director of British Medical Council Pneumoconiosis Research Unit PRU).

In 1951, three groups, PRU, France and IL0 jointly issued “Proposed Anglo-French Classification of Radiographs in Pneumoconiosis” by combining profusion with size/type referring to the 1950 ILO Classification, using three languages; for example, the current terms of small opacities were denoted as simple penumoconiosis (PRU), ombres fines (French) and pneumocniosis with discrete opacities (ILO). The concept of combining profusion with size/type may have been a basis toward later classifications (6).

The 1958 Classification

Scope: Mineral dusts

The 1950 Sydney classification was widely used, particularly in connection with coal miner's pneumoconiosis, but did not cover pneumoconioses occurring in other industries. To cope with the users' voice, ILO called another expert meeting at Geneva at the end of 1958. The experts agreed to make a single classification for various pneumoconioses provoked by mineral dusts, and entitled "the International Classification of Persistent Opacities in the Lung Field Provoked by the Inhalation of Mineral Dusts". (9) (Table 6.1)

Over 900 standard radiograph sets were distributed to 55 countries.

In this classification, profusion of small opacities was expressed by an indirect estimate of number combined with extension in the lung fields. The guidelines mentioned that "The basic idea underlying the categorization of small opacities was that of number, but as simple count was impossible, an indirect estimate of number had to be made from an unhappy combination of extension and profusion."

Table 6.1. Overview of Development of ILO Internatioanl Classification of Radiographs of Pneumoconioses

		1950	1958	1968 extended	1971	1980	2000
Small opacities (1958-)	Profusion	0 Discrete opacities 1 2 3 X(Others)	0 Z(Suspect) 1 2 3	0 (0/-, 0/0, 0/1) 1 (1/0, 1/1, 1/2) 2 (2/1, 2/2, 2/3) 3 (3/2, 3/3, 3/+)			
	Size/type	Optional code P=pinhead M=macronodular N=nodular	Small opacities p=punctiform m=micronodular n=nodular	Rounded opacities p q r			
			L=Linear /reticular	Irregular opacities s t u			
Large opacities (1958-)		Coalescent /massive A=1cm+ B C D=distortion	A B C				
Pleural abnormalities		No mention	Symbol:pl	Pleural thickening Pleural calcification Diaphragma Wall	Cost-phrenic angle Chest wall Ill-defined diaphragm pl calcification	Chest wall Diaphragama Cost-phrenic angle	Plaque Cost-phrenic angle Diffuse

Remarks: The 1968 version has two classifications; short and extended. The short one is similar to the 1958 version except for pleural abnormalities (plc and pl). The table shows only extended classification.

The 1968 Classification

Scope: mineral dusts including coal and carbon

Some experts were critical of the 1958 category 1 profusion standard film as representing profusion below a typical category 1. To meet these objections, new film selections were made of the category 1 standard (mid-category) film.

Later when a further revision of the Classification was being prepared, the International Union Against Cancer (UICC) groups gathered in Cincinnati in 1967 to propose UICC/Cincinnati Classification mainly to deal with asbestos-related lung and pleural abnormalities (10). In order to address this concern, the 1968 ILO classification included an "extended classification" to deal with asbestos-related abnormalities in addition to a "short classification" to handle mineral dusts, including coal and carbon. (11) (Table 6.2)
The "Extended classification" included the following three important changes.

1) Profusion: Each of the 4 major point scales (0, 1, 2, and 3) was further sub-divided into 3 (0/-, 0/0, 0/1 ; 1/0, 1/1, 1/2 ; 2/1, 2/2, 2/3 ; 3/2, 3/3 and 3/4) which had originally been used by the British National Coal Board. Thus, the 12 minor point scale system was adopted. (Note 3/4 was described as 3/+ in the 1980 version)

2) Irregular opacities. Irregular small opacities were classified as L in the 1958 version, but in this revision acquired three letter designations for the first time analogous to the counterpart of small rounded opacities.

3) Pleural abnormalities. Another major change was about pleural thickening and calcification. The two were to be classified before listing other symbols. Pleural abnormalities were graded, focusing on asbestos-related pleural conditions.

Table 6.2. Scopes of the ILO International Classfications of Radiographs of Pneumoconioses

1950	Mineral dusts
1958	Mineral dusts
1968	Mineral dusts including coal and carbon
1971	All types of mineral dusts, including silica, coal, asbestos, & beryllium
1980	Dusts
2000	Dusts

The 1971 Classification

Scope: All types of mineral dusts including silica, coal, asbestos and beryllium

In 1970, the ILO and UICC groups convened a joint meeting in Cardiff to publish the comprehensive classification of pneumoconioses under the name of ILO U/C International Classification of Radiographs of Pneumoconioses 1971(12). Therefore, the 1968 version had a short life of only 3 years (Table 6.1).

The main items proposed by UICC groups had already been adopted in the 1968 extended classification.

The 1980 ILO Classification

Scope: Dusts

At the 1978, ILO Geneva Meeting, the ILO expert group including the author recommended selection of new standard radiographs. Two years later, the 1980 revision of the Classification was published (13, 14) .

How the 1980 standard radiographs were selected.

The reading trial to provide the 1980 new standards was assisted scientifically and financially by US National Institute of Safety and Health (NIOSH), and American College of Radiology (ACR), though at that time USA withdrew its ILO membership. The ILO international expert group headed by George Jacobson and later Russell Morgan collected more than 200 candidate standard radiographs in cooperation with world experts. Considering the quality of films, they finally selected 106 candidate films. Then, 27 specialists; 10 Europeans, 8 Americans and 9 Japanese, read these films in reference to the 1971 standard films. The reading trial was little criticized by the method in which the films were read as they included the 1971 standards themselves. As a result, many of the 1971 standards came to be selected again. The statistical analysis of the standard film reading trial was performed initially by Harlan Amandus in the U.S. at NIOSH. Based on his data, a further study was made by T. Matsumoto and the author (15), as described below.

1) Selection of standard films. Each standard radiograph, for example the 1/1 p/p standard radiograph, was selected among from candidate radiographs whose reading variation was the smallest (Fig. 6.1).
   Likewise, the 1/1 t/t standard was determined (Fig. 6.2).
2) Reading difference in rounded and irregular small opacities (Fig. 6.3):
   Rounded small opacity profusion showed a smaller reading variation than irregular ones, especially in the low profusion categories. Furthermore, the two curves show a different upward tendency from 0/- to 3/+.

3) Middling tendency (Fig. 6.4). Out of 12 point profusion scales, only 4 major middle category films are actually available and the remaining 8 sub-categories should be mentally decided. The reading scores proved that the 3 major middle categories (1/1, 2/2, and 3/3) had a higher rate than the remaining 8 categories for which no standard radiographs were available.
4) International reading variations (Fig. 6.5): There were definite international reading variations, even though all readers referred to the same standards. That is, Japanese readers showed higher average scores of small opacity profusion than Europeans and Americans whose reading variations were nearly the same.

At a workshop of the 1988 ILO Pittsburgh Pennsylvania Conference on the Pneumoconioses users strongly demanded an effort to revise the text and attempt to select 0/1 and 1/0 boundary standards.

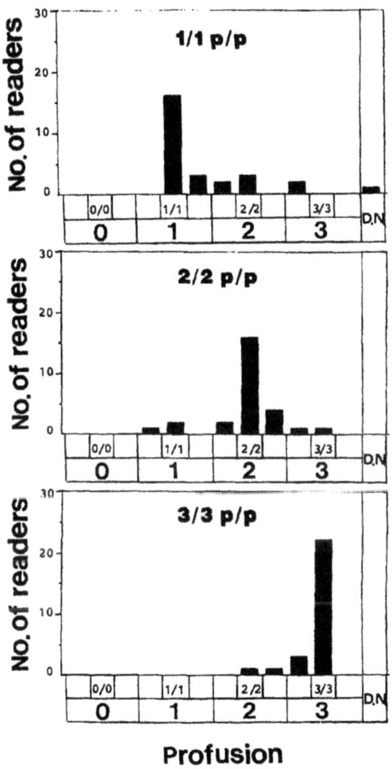

Fig. 6.1. Selection of the 1980 and 2000 standard radiographs (15). Reading variations among international experts for the 1/1 p/p standard films

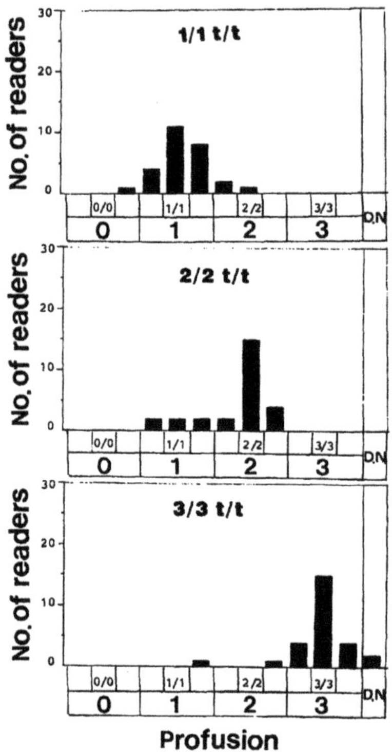

Fig. 6.2. Selection of the 1980 (2000)standard radiographs (15). Reading variations among international experts for the 1/1 t/t standard films

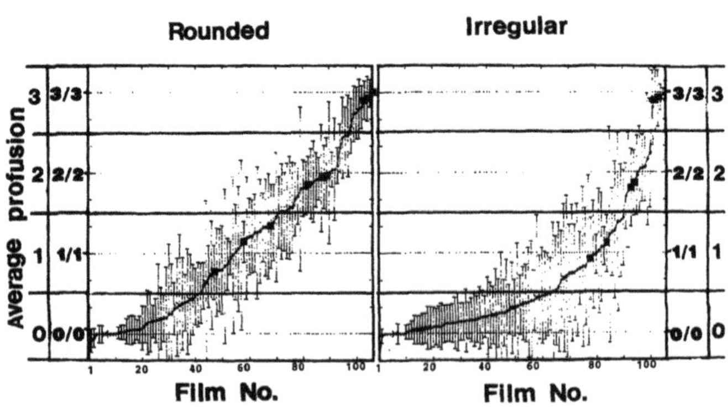

Fig. 6.3. Selection of the 1980 (2000) standard radiographs (15). Reading difference in rounded and irregular small opacities

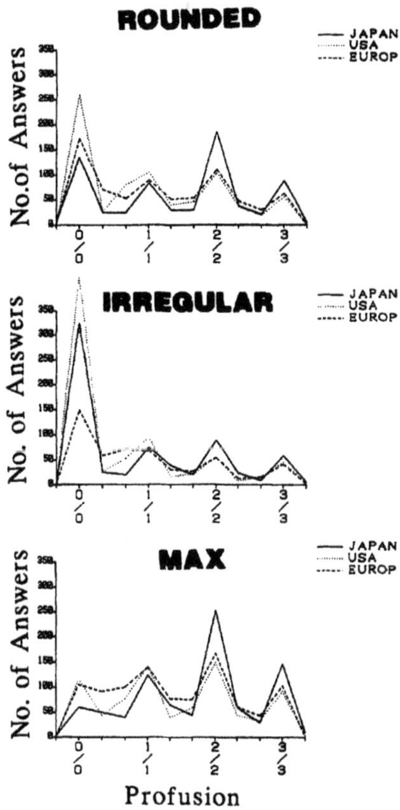

Fig. 6.4. Selection of the 1980 (2000) standard radiographs (15). Middling tendency of reading results: more in middle-categories than other minor categories

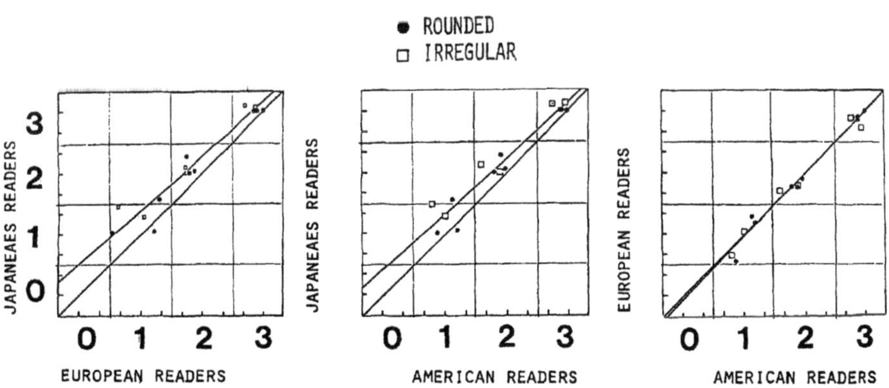

Fig. 6.5. Selection of the 1980 (2000) standard radiographs (15). Overall international reading variations between European, US and Japanese experts

Training of readers

The purpose of training is to reduce inter- and intra-observers variations and many countries have made efforts to train radiologists, occupational doctors and chest physician. In 1949, Fletcher was deeply concerned with the problem of consistent radiological diagnosis in pneumoconiosis (16). In 1970, a unique teaching method of weekend "view box seminar" was developed by American College of Radiology (ACR) to train radiologists to interpret and classify the radiological manifestations of pneumoconiosis (17). This seminar combined two pedagogic techniques, group view box study and a test-teach-test sequence of instruction that compels active participation in the learning process. Every two trainees are assigned to a long view box with enough space for 2-3 films. Those who finish the training course may be given A-reader certificates, while B-reader certificates are given to who successfully pass a test administered by NIOSH. It became evident later that even B-readers lose skills if they did not frequently interpret occupational radiographs. In 1984, a recertification examination system was introduced. To remain certified as a NIOSH B reader, an individual was required to be re-certified every 4 years or to begin the process over after a waiting period. Analysis of the pass-fail rate indicates that over-reading is a major factor in failing the examination.

Such ACR view box seminars were so far held about 40 times in US. In other countries, ACR-system view box seminars are also growing in popularity. ILO organized several ACR-system view box seminars in Asia (Vietnam, Thailand and Indonesia) by inviting ACR and Japanese instructors. Japan held two big seminars; in Kyoto in 1997 and Tsuruga in 2001 participated by about 100 trainees, in addition to the annual training course for overseas and domestic trainees in Rosai Hospital for Silicosis, Japan.

The 2000 ILO Classification

Scope: Dusts

Since the publication of the 1980 version, ILO expert group informally gathered to revise 1980 classification in various occasions in Tokyo (1983), Bochum (1983) , Nikko Japan (1988) and Pittsburgh (1988). One of the important recommendations made by them is that no change should be made in the ILO International Radiographs of Pneumocnioses until the existing evidence and views had been reviewed. This group also proposed to examine the possibility of use of sectional standards.

In 1989, ILO called an expert meeting in Geneva to review the 1980 classification. Unexpectedly, it took more than 10 years before finalizing the publication of next version, the 2000 version, because of a large-scale international reading trial of quadrant standards. It took 11 years before finalizing the millennium (2000) guidelines at the Washington DC expert meeting in December 2000.

The guidelines of the 2000 version are likely more practical than the 1980 guidelines, though the standard radiographs are the same except for sectional or quadrant films and a new film of pleural abnormalities. Film reproduction technique was changed to digital copy style.

Quadrant standard radiographs

For the use of standard radiographs, x-ray readers are always requested to read films in reference to standard radiographs, not using mental images of standards that are in readers' mind. However, it is an actually troublesome work for readers to compare a film to be read with several category standards whenever they read. Already in the 1970s, experienced radiologists such as Russell Morgan were using a home-made composite (sectional) standard radiograph (quadrant or sextant on a radiograph) . The Japanese Ministry of Labour officially adopted quadrant standards ahead of the international use, based on the domestic reading trial (18).

An ILO expert group made a large-scale trial for the use of quadrant radiographs, aiming to establish whether and to what extent, use of composite standard radiographs would affect readers' classifications of chest films in persons who have been exposed occupationally to dust. Thirty-nine physicians from 10 countries joined the study to repeatedly classify 120 chest radiographs in reference to full size and quadrant standards (19).

The summary and conclusions were based on 12,929 valid film reading sheets by 39 readers and are as follows:

The proposed modification to the ILO standard radiographs, involving reproductions of sections from 15 of the ILO standards on five new quadrant films,

1) would not increase variability between readers, and might improve reproducibility of small opacity profusion classifications in some respects
2) but could also reduce slightly the frequency with which some readers identify large opacities
3) is likely to increase the frequency with which some readers describe the shapes of the small opacities that they see as predominantly irregular rather than rounded.

Classification of small opacity profusion for films identified as predominantly irregular are likely to be higher using the modified standards when compared to the same classification using the current ILO 1980 full-size standards.

The results were detectable in the context of a controlled trial setting, involving a contrived high proportion of films classifiable as showing small opacities (about 60% with category 1 or more). The effects described are unlikely to be distinguishable from *inter- and intra-* reader variability in most real-life occupational health survey situation where the prevalence of pneumoconiosis is usually less severe.

Thus, use of the quadrant standard film sets was recommended by the expert group of the ILO. Indeed, the ILO has now issued Quadrant or Composite Standard films along with the Full-size Standard films.

Future Aspects of ILO Classification

Radiographic techniques

The current standard radiographs were taken with traditional analog-system of conventional film-screen method. A great disadvantage of analog system x-rays is that images of radiographs with both side emulsion are aging with time and it is difficult to keep the original quality and they deteriorate over time, even with good storage conditions. In case of digital radiography, no such decay occurs. The 1980 ILO standard films are photo-printed copies of the analog radiographs. When the ILO experts compared the photo-printed standard films with digitally acquired films at a Washington Meeting on in 2000, they agreed that digital ones were superior to photo-copied ones. Eventually, both x-ray-taking and copying techniques will change to digital methods. The ILO has been encouraged to provide a collection of digital standard radiographs of good quality to be copied by digital techniques for the next version.

Size of chest radiographs

Almost all images by CT, isotope study, MRI and ultrasound are obtained in reduced size, and not full life size. Only the conventional film-screen system gives life size images. A study revealed that reduced size computed chest radiographs (1/2 in length, or 1/4 in area) provide similar reading results when compared with the reduced size standards (19). With the wide use of digital images, digital radiographs will be read on CRT or liquid crystal display and not on view boxes and not in full life size. Ultimately, it will not be possible and indeed there will be no reason to continue the use of full or life size images.

Computed tomography

Recently CT has become an indispensable tool to examine pulmonary parenchymal and pleural abnormalities, because of the shortened exposure time (as long as 20 seconds was required in the late 1970s) (21) and lowered radiation exposure. With the resolution of these problems, CT came to be used even for the screening purpose in some countries such as Finland and Germany. With frequent CT use, an international CT classification has been proposed. Initially, researchers tried to make an HRCT classification system comparable to the ILO classification, but actually the system (International Classification of HRCT for Occupational and Environmental Respiratory Diseases) is a hybrid with mixed principles of ILO chest radiographic classification system and with CT characteristic language and images. The mobile CT unit (on car) (22) will promote wider use of CT in the early diagnosis of pneumoconiosis and other lung diseases.

Acknowledgement

I acknowledge with gratitude kind help of William Jones Williams, Professor Emeritus, University of Cardiff and Mr Otha Linton, Executive Director, International Society of Radiology.

References

1) Boehme A. (1925) Die Prognose der Staublungeerkrankung (Silikose) Beitr. Klin.Tuberk, 84, 119-139
2) Pancoast HK, Pendergrass EP (1931) A review of pneumoconiosis, further roentgenological and pathological studies. A J Roentgenol, 26, 556-614
3) Gerland LH (1936), Radiology, 27, 21-32
4) Fletcher CM,Mann KJ, Davies I, Cochrane AL, Gilson JC, Hugh-Jones, J Faculty (1949)Radiologists, 1, 40-60
5) Fletcher CM, Oldham PD, (1951)The ue of standard films in the radiological diagnosis of coalworkers' pneumoconiosis, Brit J Industr Med, , 8, 138-149
6) Cochrane AL, Davies I, Fletcher CM, "entente radiologique" (1951) A step towards international agreement of the classification of radiographs in pneumoconiosis, Brit. J Industr Med, 8, 244-255
7) Fletcher CM and Oldham PD(1949), The problem of consistent radiological diagnosis in coalminers' pneumoconiosis. an experimental study Brit J Industr Med, 6, 168-183
8) Industrial Pulmonary Diseases , a symposium held at the postgraduate medical school of London 18th-20th September 1957 and 25th-27th 1958 edited by King EJ and Fletcher CM, (1960)J & A Church Hill Ltd London
9) International Labour Office, Meeting of experts on the international classification of radiographs of the pneumoconioses, Occup Safety and Health, (1959), IX, 2, April-June
10) Bohlig H, Bristol LJ, Cartier PH et al (1970), UICC/Cincinnati classification of the radiographic appearances of pneumoconioses, a cooperative study by the UICC committee Chest, 58,1, 57-67
11) International Labour Office, Inernational classification of radiographs of radiographs of pneumoconioses (revised, 1968)
12) International Labour Office, ILO/UC international classification of radiographs of pneumoconioses 1971 Occupational Safety and Health series 22 (rev)
13) Guidelines for the use of ILO international classification of radiographs of pneumoconioses, revised edition 1980, Occupational Safety and Health series 22(rev.80)
14) Hosoda Y, Shida H, Hiraga Y, (1991) Pneumoconioses in developing countries, diagnosis and management, ed Sharma OP Mecel Dekker Inc. New York,423-448
15) Matsumoto T, Fukuhisa K, Iinuma TA et al (1990) Specifications for selecting the ILO 1980 standard radiographs of pneumoconioses. A re-analysis of data obtained from an international film reading trial. Intra-mural report to the Jpn Committee for quantitative x-ray diagnosis of pneumocniosis..
16) Fletcher CM and Oldham PD(1949) The problem of consistent radiological diagnosis in coalminers' pneumoconiosis—An experimental study Brit J indust Med,6,168-183
17) Wiot JF, Linton OW (2000), The radiologist and occupational lung disease: an appeal for continued involvement Am J Radiol, 311-313
18) Hosoda Y, Shida H, Mikami R et al (1983), A stduy of the use of sectional standard radiographs of pneumoconioses In: VIth International Pneumoconiosis Conference , Vol 1 306-314 (ed Bergbau-Berufsgenossenshaft, Bochum)

19) Jacobsen M, Miller WE, Parker JE, (1997) A trial of additional composite standard radiographs for use with the ILO international classification of radiographs of pneumoconioses, NIH
20) Fukuhisa K, Iinuma TA, Matsumoto T et al (1984), Digital x-ray images of pneumoconoses and their evaluation In: Computed Radiography(ed Taeno Y, Iinuma T & Takano M) Springer-Verlag Tokyo, 175-185
21) Hosoda Y, Saito N, Hachiya T et al(1980), Differential diagnosis of asbestos-induced pleural thickening using computer tomography: A preliminary study. In: Biological Effects of Mineral Fibres Vol 2, IARC Scientific Publications No 30, , 527-536
22) Matsumoto T, Miyamoto T, Suzuki T et al(1997). Development of mobile CT unit for lung cancer. In: Advances of occupational respiratory diseases (ed. Chiyotani K, Hosoda Y, Aizawa Y) , Elsevier Science BV, 485-489

Part III

CT Images

Chapter 7 Pleural Diseases

Michael Crane [1], Pierre Alain Gevenois [2], and Marc Letourneux [3]

[1] Radiology Department, Llandough Hospital, Penlan Road, Near Penarth, Glamorgan CF64 2XX, Wales, U.K.

[2] Department of Radiology, Hospital Erasme, Universite Libre de Bruxelles, Route de Leinnik, 808 1070, Bruxelles, Belgium

[3] Service de Medecine du Travail et Pathologie Professionnelle, Niveau 1, CHU Cote de Nacre, 14033 Caen Cedex, France

Whilst many occupational and environmental diseases affect the lung parenchyma it is only asbestos dust which results in radiographic manifestations in the pleura and these may be due to either benign or malignant processes.

Benign Asbestos Induced Pleural Disease

Inhaled Asbestos fibres can induce various benign lesions of the pleura : parietal pleural plaques, visceral pleural thickening (a term that is preferred to that of "diffuse" pleural thickening), and benign pleural effusion.

Pathogenesis

The pathogenesis of these lesions remains speculative, even if the presence of asbestos fibres, found in limited areas of the parietal pleura called "black spots" by Boutin (Boutin et al. 1996), suggests the migration of inhaled fibres through the lung to the pleura, predominantly by the lymphatic pathway. The mechanisms leading to pleural plaques rather than to benign pleural effusion are not clear, but visceral pleural thickening seems to be most likely the consequence of asymptomatic benign pleural effusion (Epler et al. 1982) (Mc Loud et al. 1985) (Lilis et al. 1988).

Pathologic findings

Pleural plaques are elevated, hard ivory-coloured structures, generally bilateral, placed most typically on the parietal pleura, following the ribs, and the domes of the diaphragm. Their thickness may vary from a few mm to more than 1 cm, and their surface is free of adhesions with the adjacent visceral pleura. Microscopically, they are made of a basket weave pattern of collagen (Greenberg 1992) (Churg 1998).

Visceral pleural thickening is a non specific fibrous thickening involving the visceral pleura, consisting of dense collagenous tissue containing inflammatory cells. It is often unilateral, and may be associated with pulmonary rounded atelectasis where the pleura is drawn into the underlying atelectatic lung (Greenberg 1992).

Benign asbestos pleural effusion is an exudate and may be hemorrhagic, with non specific fibrotic lesions of the pleura.

Epidemiology

The prevalence of pleural plaques is dependent on the radiographic criteria used (Greene et al. 1984). In the United States, a prevalence rate of 3% has been reported in the general population (Rogan et al. 1987), whereas prevalence rates in asbestos-exposed occupational settings may exceed 50%. Household contacts of asbestos factory workers have shown prevalence rates up to 20% (Epler et al. 1980) (Sider et al. 1987). There does not seem to be a threshold in the dose-response relationship between asbestos exposure and pleural plaques, and this is consistent with the report of endemic pleural plaques in various geographic areas characterised by fibrous mineral outcrops (Bignon 1989) (Hiraoka et al. 1998).

In contrast with pleural plaques, the latency of which is usually over 20 years, benign pleural effusion and visceral pleural thickening may occur within the 10 years following the onset of exposure. Their prevalence is lower than that of pleural plaques (Scwartz 1991), and they are associated with higher levels of asbestos exposure (De Vuyst et al. 1998) (Rockoff et al. 1987) (Jakobsson et al. 1995).

The prevalence of pleural plaques increases with increasing time since the first exposure, but there is no clear relationship between cumulative asbestos exposure and the extent of pleural plaques (Van Cleemput et al. 2001). The possible relationship between plaque size and pulmonary function is also controversial. Various radiographic studies, some recent (Wang et al. 2001) suggest an association between pleural changes and functional pulmonary impairment, and a relationship between reduction in lung volumes and radiographic score of pleural lesions has been reported (Schwartz et al. 1990) (Broderick et al. 1992). Yet when computed tomography is performed, a more accurate differentiation between pleural plaques and visceral pleural thickening becomes possible. Then, if visceral pleural thickening proves to be related to decrease of pulmonary function parameters, pleural plaques alone appear to be not functionally relevant (Van Cleemput et al. 2001) (Copley et al. 2001).

No clear relationship has been established between pleural plaques and mesothelioma or bronchial carcinoma (Weiss 1993).

Clinical features

Most patients with pleural plaques alone are asymptomatic, and the presence of a pulmonary functional impairment raises the question of an associated parenchymal fibrosis which may be radiographically inapparent.

Chest pain and dyspnea may be present in the case of extensive visceral pleural thickening, and functional impairment can then manifest as restriction in lung volumes, independently of any radiographic sign of parenchymal fibrosis (Schwartz et al. 1990) (Rosenstock et al. 1988). Once it has appeared, this deficit in lung function does not seem to change very much over time even though the radiographic score may increase (Yates et al. 1996).

Benign pleural effusions are frequently asymptomatic, but chest pain or dyspnea are possible, and recurrence may be seen (Hillerdal and Özesmi 1987). The diagnosis of asbestos-related benign pleural effusion should not be made unless all other cause of pleural effusion has been ruled out by thoracoscopic procedures, and a negative follow-up of at least three years.

Radiological features

Pleural plaques

On postero-anterior chest radiography, pleural plaques are best observed when viewed tangentially : they then appear as focal areas of pleural thickening along the lateral chest walls, between the sixth and ninth ribs, and along the diaphragm, generally sparing the apices and the costophrenic angles. Usually bilateral, pleural plaques can also be unilateral (Koskinen et al. 1998) (Gevenois et al. 1998). They are sharply demarcated on all sides and particularly from the lungs. When viewed en face, they may appear as hazy densities, more visible when enhanced by calcification (Greenberg 1992)(Fig. 7.1). Their extent in length and in thickness can be assessed according to the ILO Classification of Radiographs of Pneumoconioses (International Labour Office 1980).

A high false negative radiographic detection rate has been reported in autopsy studies : small plaques on the anterior or posterior chest wall, or on the diaphragm, are particularly difficult to detect by standard chest films (Greenberg 1992). Conversely, false positive diagnosis can result from misinterpretation of sub pleural fat pad or extrapleural muscles. Oblique radiographs have been proposed in order to increase sensitivity of detection (Baker and Greene 1982), but they also tend to enhance false positive rate and are not recommended (Ameille and al. 1993).

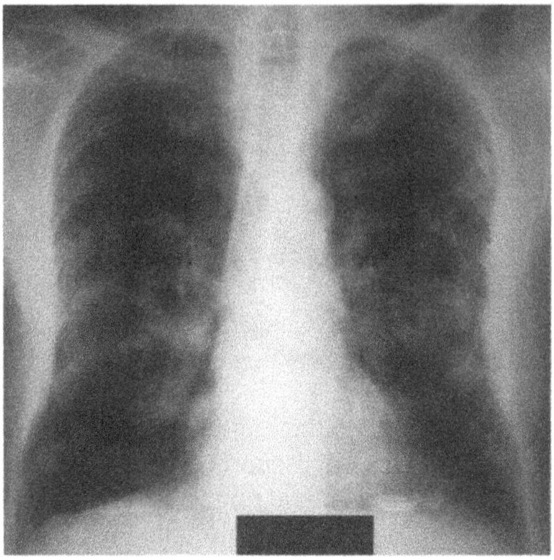

Fig. 7.1. Plain chest radiograph : bilateral calcified pleural plaques are viewed en face and on the diaphragm

CT of the thorax has been shown to increase both sensitivity and specificity for the detection of pleural plaques (Aberle et al. 1988) (Friedman et al. 1988) (Al Jarad et al. 1991). Pleural plaques are recognized as focal areas of pleural thickening, with solid attenuation values and sometimes including calcifications. They may have a typical tableland shape (Fig. 7.2) or be a flat thickening of the pleura (Fig. 7.3); what defines their parietal nature are their smooth and sharply defined edges, well demarcated from adjacent extrapleural tissues on one hand, and from adjacent lung on the other hand. Their attenuation values are different from those of extrapleural fat deposits (Fig. 7.4), and CT scan can also show them when they are located on the diaphragm (Fig. 7.5).

A focal stripe of parenchymal ground glass opacity can sometimes be seen next to thick parietal pleural plaques, at a small distance from the pleural thickening ; probably a consequence of focal alveolar collapse.

The frequent location of pleural plaques in paraspinal regions of the thorax is easily identified by CT (Fig. 7.3 and Fig. 7.5), but sometimes intercostal vessels mimicking pleural thickening need to be recognised (Fig. 7.6); the presence of thickening on multiple levels, the visibility of extrapleural fat between the pleura and intercostal vessels, or the presence of calcification within the abnormality, may help to identify the pleural origin of the opacity (Im et al. 1989).

In subjects with only "passive exposure" to asbestos, such as living or working in a building with known asbestos contamination, a CT study has reported minor pleural changes. The significance of these changes is unknown because of the poor inter-observer agreement in this study, and because of the lack of histopathologic confirmation (De Raeve et al. 2001).

Even if the pathologic meaning of very subtle pleural changes may sometimes be unclear, CT allows the identification of small parietal pleural plaques measuring no more than 1 or 2 mm in thickness on the chest wall. They can be differentiated from the normal intercostal stripe which includes the thickness of normal visceral and parietal pleurae, the endothoracic fascia, and the innermost intercostal muscle (Fig. 7.7). In paravertebral regions, where intercostal muscles are absent, even a thin stripe can be consistent with asbestos-related pleural thickening (Webb et al. 1996).

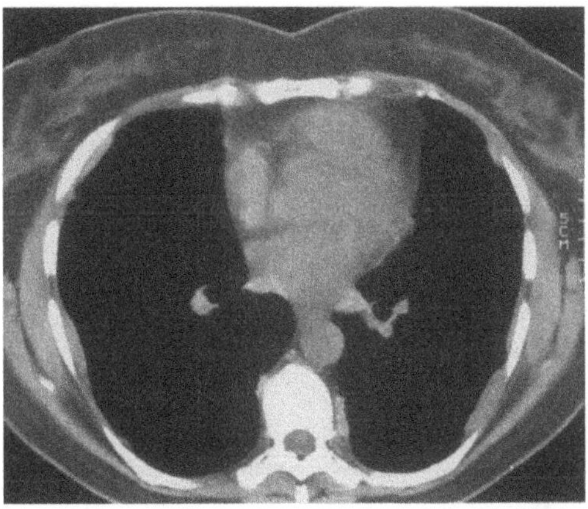

Fig. 7.2. CT scan : typical tableland shaped bilateral pleural plaques

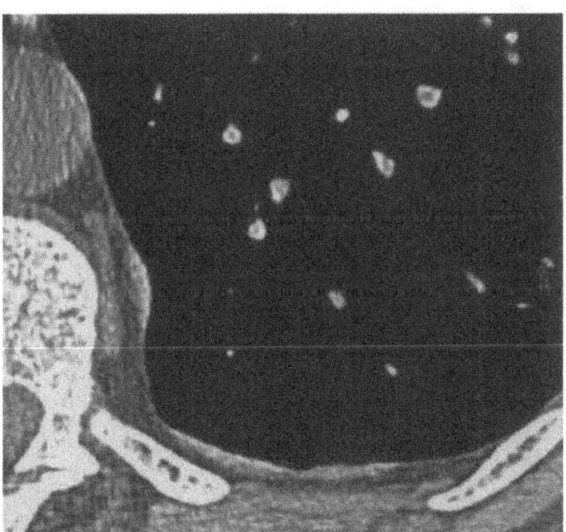

Fig. 7.3. CT scan : pleural plaques with tapering margins

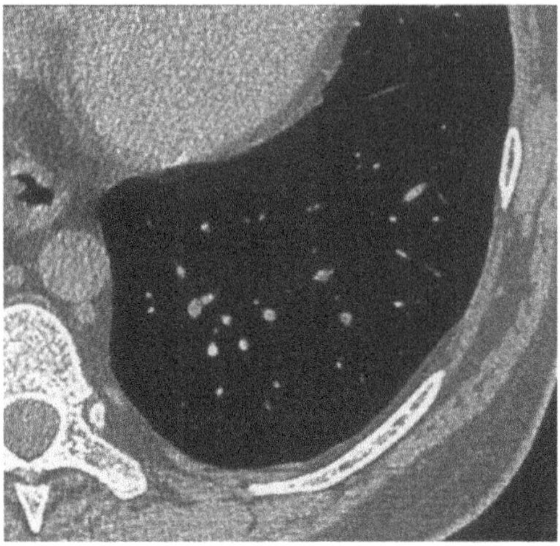

Fig. 7.4. CT scan : subpleural fat deposit

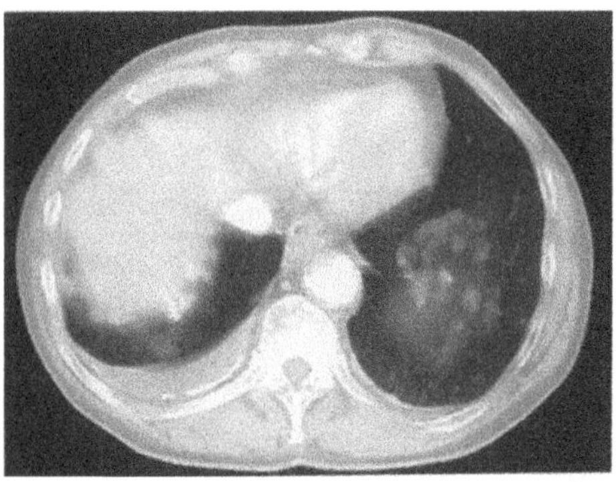

Fig. 7.5. CT scan : pleural plaques are visible on the diaphragm, with calcification on the right side. Bilateral calcified pleural plaques can also be seen on the parietal pleura, and a right pleural effusion is present

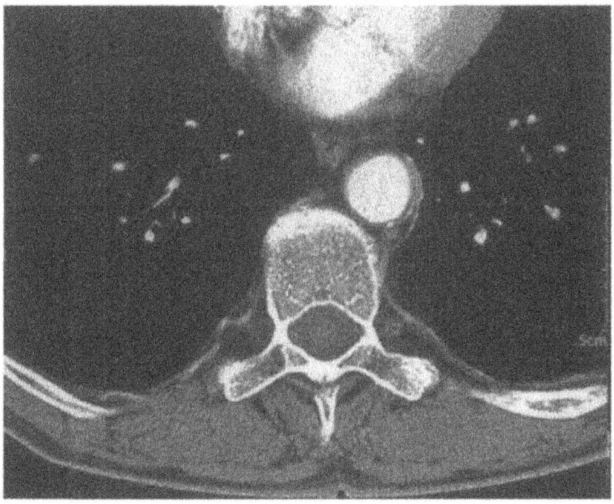

Fig. 7.6. CT scan : intercostal vessels in paraspinal regions of the thorax

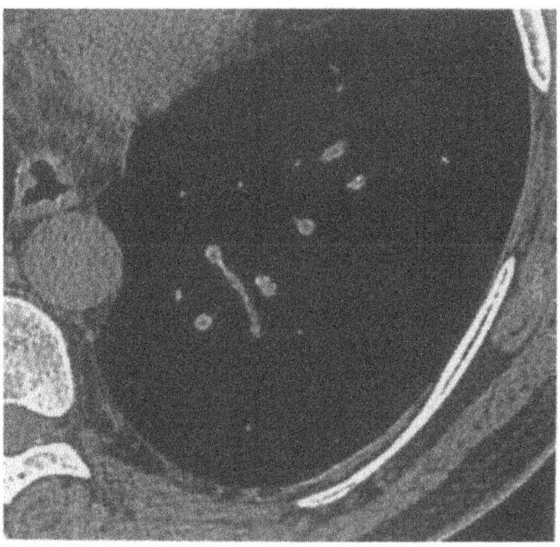

Fig. 7.7. CT scan : normal intercostal stripe

Mild diaphragmatic pleural changes may be more difficult to recognise.

In some patients the transversus thoracis muscle and subcostalis muscle must be differentiated from pleural plaques. Adjacent to the lower sternum or the xiphoïd process, the transversus thoracis muscles are often visible internal to the anterior ends of ribs or costal cartilage. Subcostalis muscles may rarely be present, at the same level, along the posterior chest wall, internal to one or more ribs (Webb et al. 1996) (Fig. 7.8).

In subjects with silicosis, or in the case of other pulmonary granulomatous diseases, confluent sub-pleural parenchymal nodules can mimic parietal pleural thickening ("pseudo-plaques") (Fig. 7.9).

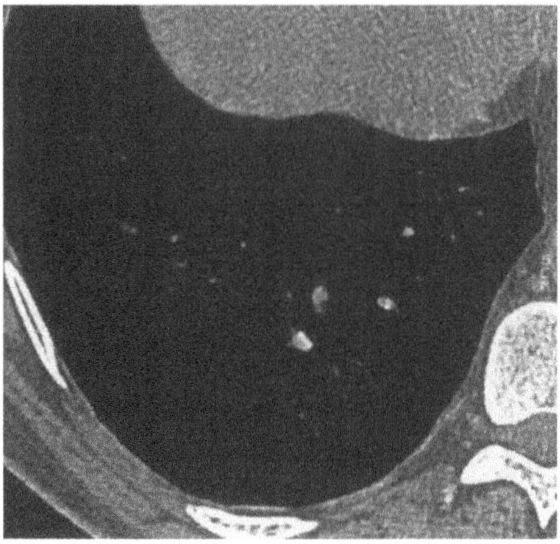

Fig. 7.8. CT scan : subcostalis muscle

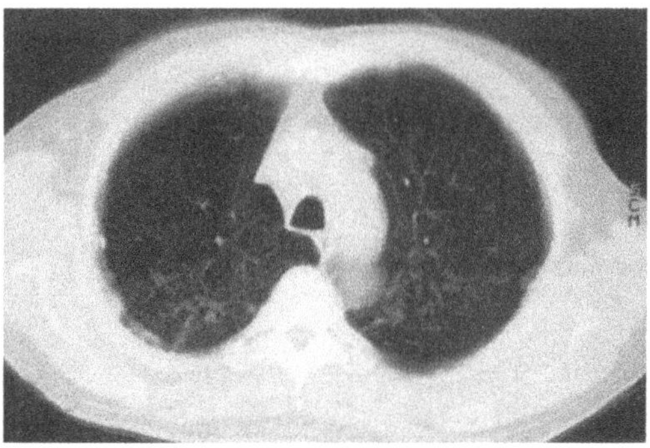

Fig. 7.9. CT scan : confluent subpleural pulmonary nodules mimicking parietal pleural thickening

Visceral pleural thickening

The radiographic appearance of so-called diffuse pleural thickening has been defined as smooth non interrupted pleural density extending over at least one quarter of the chest wall, internal to the lower ribs, with or without costophrenic angle obliteration (Mc Loud et al. 1985) (Fig. 7.10). Differentiation from pleural plaques remains difficult, and the revised edition of the ILO Classification does not eliminate some uncertainty (International Labour Office 1980). Sargent *et al.* proposed to reserve the term diffuse pleural thickening to pleural thickening associated with homolateral costophrenic angle obliteration, (Sargent et al. 1978). This restrictive definition had the merit of clarifying the radiographic diagnosis, but could not account for possible focal visceral thickening without costophrenic angle obliteration.

A CT definition of diffuse pleural thickening relying only on dimensional criteria has previously been proposed (Lynch et al. 1989). This did not take into account the possibility of widely extended pleural plaques.

The major discriminative feature of visceral pleural thickening is that the adjacent lung parenchyma is usually affected by the pleural disease, and this is manifested by parenchymal bands and rounded atelectasis.

Parenchymal bands are linear opacities 2-5 cm length, sometimes shorter, extending from the pleural thickening through the lung. They may be visible on a plain PA chest radiograph (Fig. 7.11) and, on CT of the thorax, they appear as coarse linear opacities, with a tapering shape and a course different from that of vessels (Fig. 7.12). When they radiate from the surface of the pleural thickening, they can give the appearance of "crows' feet" (Hillerdal 1985).

Although situated in the lung, rounded atelectasis must be mentioned among pleural diseases because it is always associated with a visceral pleural thickening.

Rounded atelectasis is due to lung folding at the thickened pleural surface, and is particularly seen in the lingula, middle lobe, or lower lobes (Hillerdal 1989).

It is frequently associated with parenchymal bands, and is sometimes visible on plain X-rays as a rounded opacity that may be confused with lung cancer (Payne et al. 1980).

On CT scans of the thorax, rounded atelectasis is generally easily recognised as it contacts with a thickened pleura and the bronchovascular structures sweep into the mass with a comet tail appearance (Mc Hugh and Blaquiere 1989) associated with a volume loss of adjacent lung (Lynch et al. 1988) (Gevenois et al. 1994) (Fig. 7.13).

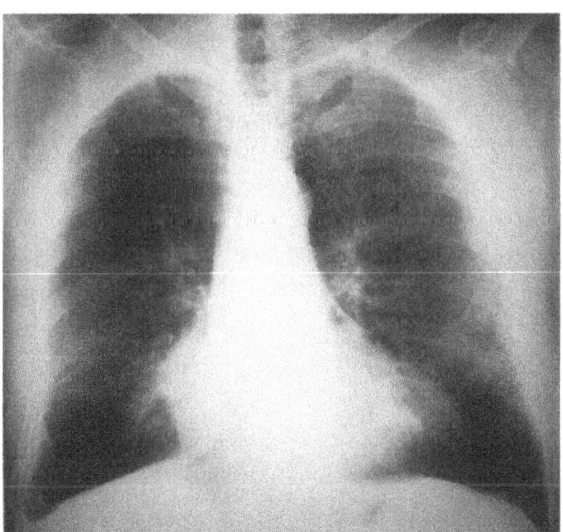

Fig. 7.10. Plain chest radiograph : bilateral pleural thickening with a visceral (or diffuse) type on the right side (costophrenic angle obliteration)

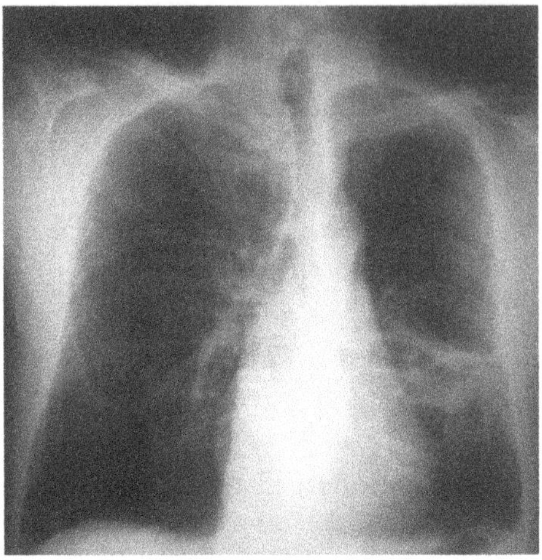

Fig. 7.11. Plain chest radiograph : left visceral pleural thickening, with costophrenic angle obliteration and parenchymal bands

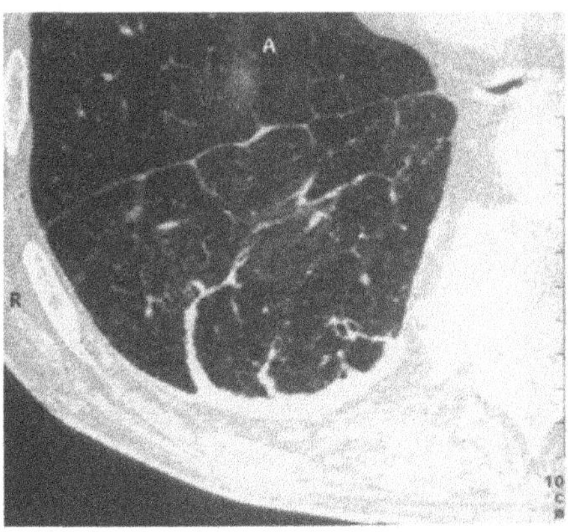

Fig. 7.12. CT scan : visceral pleural thickening with parenchymal bands ; a fissural pleural thickening is also present

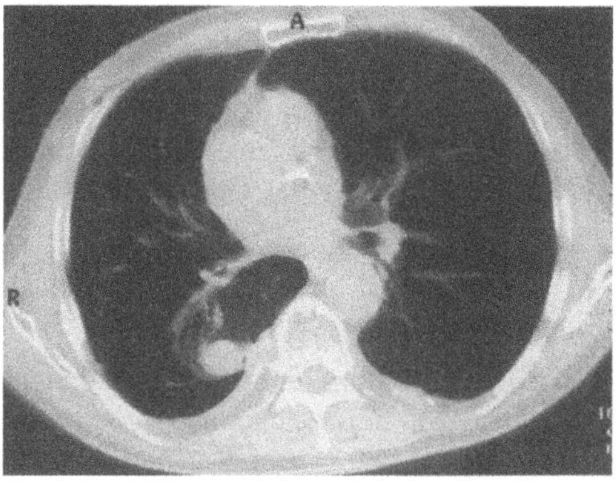

Fig. 7.13. CT scan : right rounded atelectasis

In a population of asbestos-exposed workers with normal or near-normal radiographs, PA Gevenois clearly identified visceral pleural fibrosis as a distinct pattern from pleural plaques or pulmonary fibrosis (Gevenois et al. 1998).

So whatever the extent of the pleural changes, visceral pleural thickening should be diagnosed as soon as pleural thickening, even if circumscribed, and even with non tapering margins, is associated with parenchymal bands with or without rounded atelectasis. Observation of "hairy plaques" is not unusual, and such abnormalities should be classified among visceral changes, that is visceral pleural thickening. Conversely, widely extended pleural thickening, free of any parenchymal shadowing such as parenchymal bands or rounded atelectasis, should be classified as pleural plaques even when its margins have a tapered shape (Fig. 7.3).

Visceral pleural thickening may exist in the absence of any pulmonary fibrosis, but, when pulmonary asbestosis is present, parenchymal changes adjacent to pleural thickening may be difficult to interpret, and definition of the strictly parietal or visceral type of the pleural thickening may be uncertain.

Pleural calcification can occur in visceral pleural thickening as well as in pleural plaques (Aberle et al. 1988).

Circumscribed pleural thickening can rarely be localised in a fissure and the position within the line of the fissure will help to rule out a pulmonary origin for the opacity.

Benign pleural effusion

There is no specific radiographic or tomodensitometric feature for asbestos-related benign pleural effusion.

Computed tomography of the thorax may reveal a higher attenuation value in the case of a hemorrhagic effusion, and tomodensitometry can also be useful in order to exclude pleural effusions of pulmonary origin (Solomon 1991).

Diffuse Malignant Mesothelioma

Diffuse mesothelioma was an uncommon tumour in the early 1970's but there has been a relentless increase in annual deaths from the disease since that time (Rudd 1995) (Ferguson et al. 1987) and the incidence is expected to increase until 2020 (Pieto et al. 1995).

Exposure to asbestos is by far the most important risk factor for the development of this neoplasm (Whitwell and Rawcliffe 1971) (Teta 1983) (Edge and Choudhury 1978).

Incidence figures vary considerably in different regions and this largely reflects the likelihood of asbestos exposure whether that be occupational or environmental. The majority of mesotheliomas occur in men (Lamphear and Buncher 1992) and this reflects occupational asbestos exposure. The mean age at diagnosis is between 60 and 65 years.

Radiological features

Plain chest radiographs typically demonstrate a unilateral nodular or lobulated thickening of the pleura which may be localised or extend such that it encases the lung. The tumour may be seen extending along the line of the interlobar fissures (Brenner et al. 1982).

There maybe an accompanying pleural effusion which can vary from a small amount up to a large volume which obscures the underlying tumour. Lung encasement may fix the mediastinum such that the shift is less than with other causes of a large effusion.

The affected hemithorax may show evidence of loss of volume and this may be very marked. Calcification of the tumour is rare but reported.

In advanced tumours chest wall invasion may be identified by rib erosion, destruction or periosteal reaction. Haematogenous metastases to the lungs may be seen as multiple nodules or masses. Rarely a miliary or an interstitial pattern is identified (Fraser et al. 1999) (Solomons et al. 1985) (Ohishi et al. 1996)

CT findings

When mesothelioma is suspected or considered a possible diagnosis the CT scan would usually be performed with a volumetric technique and contiguous image slices; a high resolution technique is not likely to be utilised in usual clinical practice. CT shows the presence and extent of the tumour with greater accuracy than plain films and it demonstrates the accompanying pleural fluid with greater sensitivity (Law et al. 1982).

On CT the soft tissue density of the tumour can be readily distinguished from the adjacent pleural fluid (Fig. 7.14). Frequently the pleural thickening is extensive and gross but on occasions apparently not marked although the tumour is frequently more extensive at the time of operation than predicted from the immediate pre-operative CT scan. The mediastinal pleura can be thickened (Fig. 7.15). Unilateral pleural effusions are identified at presentation in between 30% and 80% of cases. When the tumour encases the lung the hemithorax is frequently contracted (Fig. 7.16). CT frequently demonstrates extension of the tumour into a major or less commonly a minor fissure (Alexander et al. 1981) (Müller 1993). Rarely a mesothelioma is seen on CT presenting as a solitary mass. Calcification within mesotheliomas is seen in approximately 10% of cases and usually represents engulfment of benign asbestos induced plaques (Kawashima and Libshitz 1990) (Fig. 7.17). Rarely it is the result of an osteosarcomatous component.

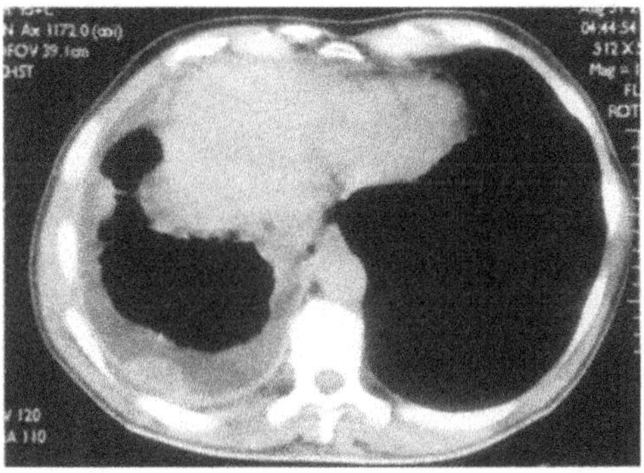

Fig. 7.14. CT scan: 66 year old man with sarcomatous mesothelioma. There is a right pleural effusion, diffuse thickening of the parietal pleura but also a localised well defined tumour mass

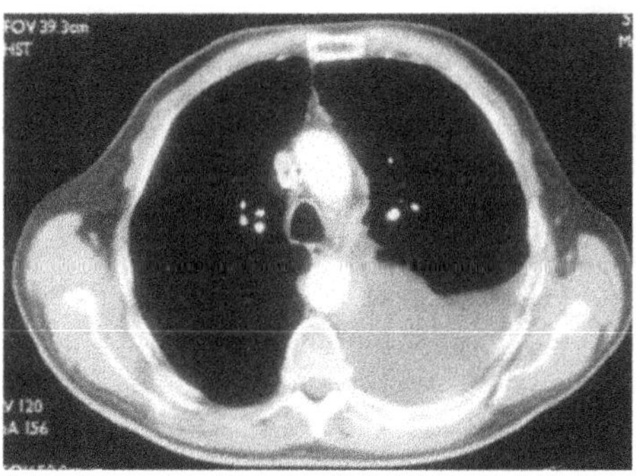

Fig. 7.15. CT scan: 78 year old man with a histologically proven mesothelioma. There is a left pleural effusion and there is irregular thickening of the mediastinal pleura overlying the ascending aorta. There is no shift of the mediastinum

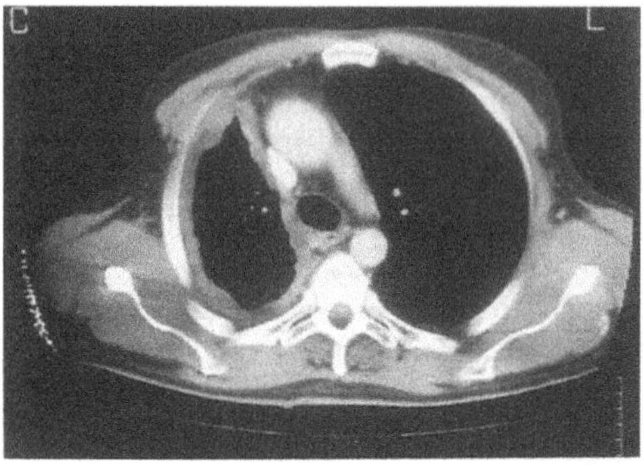

Fig. 7.16. CT scan: 49 year old man with histologically proven mesothelioma. The right lung is encircled by nodular pleural thickening and there is contraction of the right hemithorax

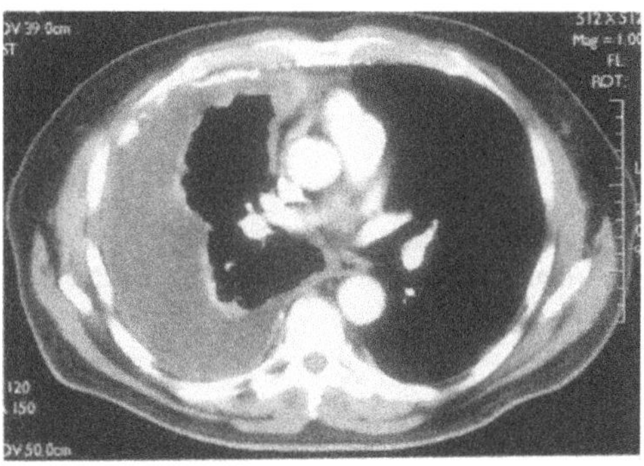

Fig. 7.17. CT scan: 72 year old man with epithelioid mesothelioma. There is a large right pleural effusion with thickening of both visceral and parietal pleura with areas of calcification due to engulfment of pre-existing benign plaques

CT is superior to conventional radiography in the assessment of invasion of the mediastinum, chest wall and upper abdomen (Alexander et al. 1981).

Findings suggesting chest wall invasion include indistinct fat planes, infiltration of intercostal muscles (Fig. 7.18), periosteal reaction and bone destruction (Fig. 7.19).

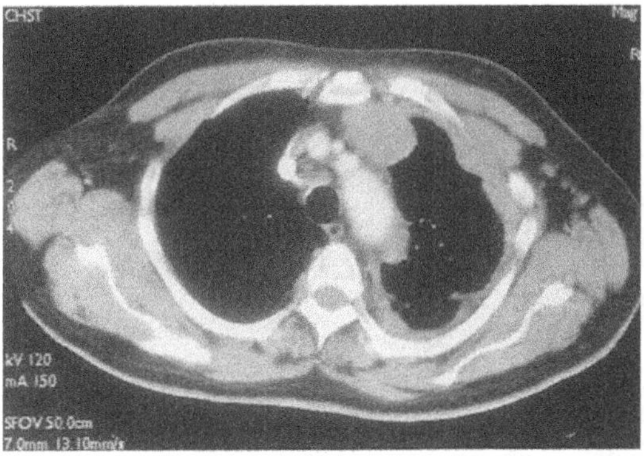

Fig. 7.18. CT scan: 68 year old man with an epithelial mesothelioma. The soft tissue tumour is seen encircling the left lung including extension over the mediastinal pleural surface. There is direct invasion of the tumour into the soft tissues of the chest wall anteriorly. The patient complained of localised chest wall pain at this site. There are enlarged nodes in the pre tracheal region

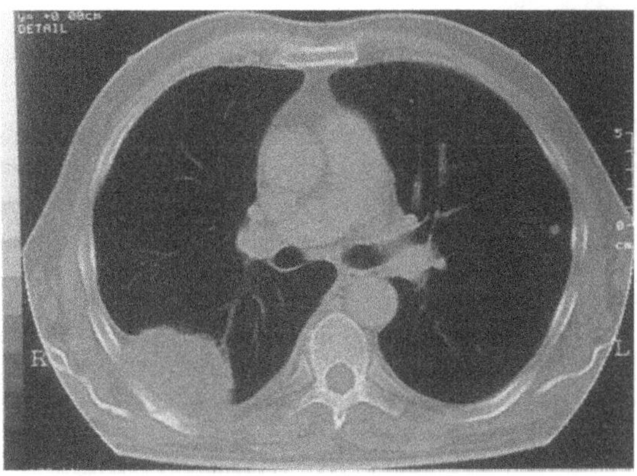

Fig. 7.19. CT scan: 45 year old man with proven a histologically proven mesothelioma. There is a localised mass in the right hemithorax postero-laterally with evidence of rib destruction and a metastasis is noted in the left lung

Features of mediastinal invasion include obscuration of fat planes, nodular or diffuse pericardial thickening (Fig. 7.20) and direct soft tissue invasion (Fig. 7.21).

Enlarged lymph nodes are not infrequently seen (Fig. 7.22). Extension of the tumour to the contra-lateral thoracic cavity is not uncommon in advanced cases. The tumour may invade through the diaphragm into the upper abdomen (Alexander et al. 1981) (Fig. 7.23). Extension of the tumour outside of the pleural cavity is seen in approximately 11% of patients at presentation, increasing to over 50% during the course of the disease (Brenner et al. 1982) (Mirvis et al. 1983).

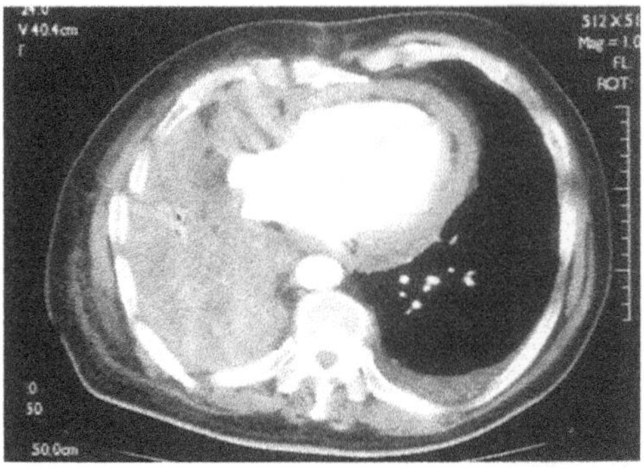

Fig. 7.20. CT scan: 65 year old man with a biphasic mesothelioma. There is an extensive bulky tumour mass within the right hemithorax which is slightly contracted. The tumour has invaded the pericardium which shows diffuse thickening. There is a small left pleural effusion

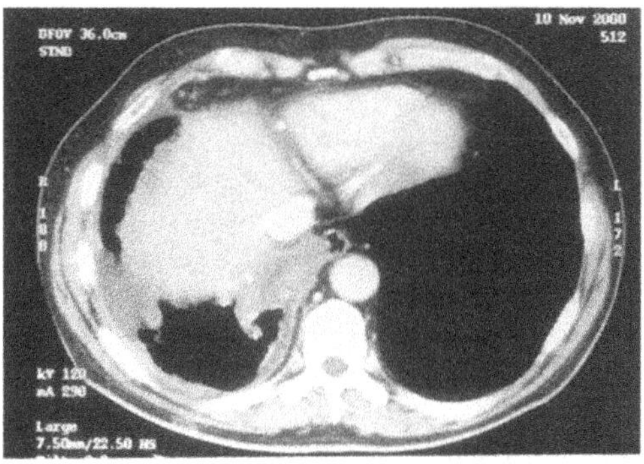

Fig. 7.21. CT scan: 59 year old man with an epithelial mesothelioma. There is thickening of both parietal and visceral pleura with a small right pleural effusion. The tumour has directly invaded the mediastinum and a mass is seen adjacent to the right wall of the oesophagus

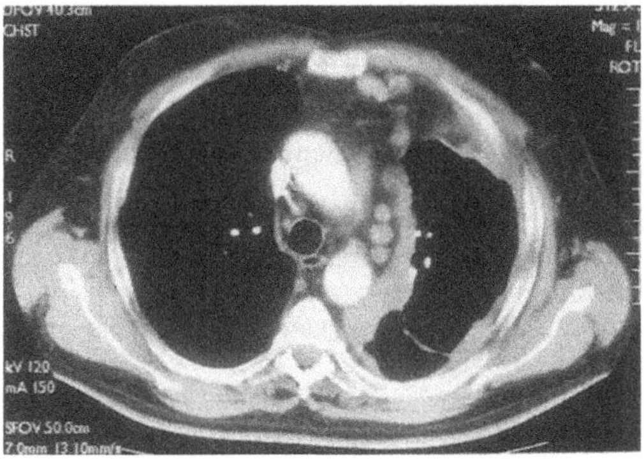

Fig. 7.22. CT scan: 69 year old man with an epithelial mesothelioma. Left sided tumour with thickening of both costal and mediastinal pleura. Several enlarged nodes are seen in the mediastinum adjacent to the aortic arch

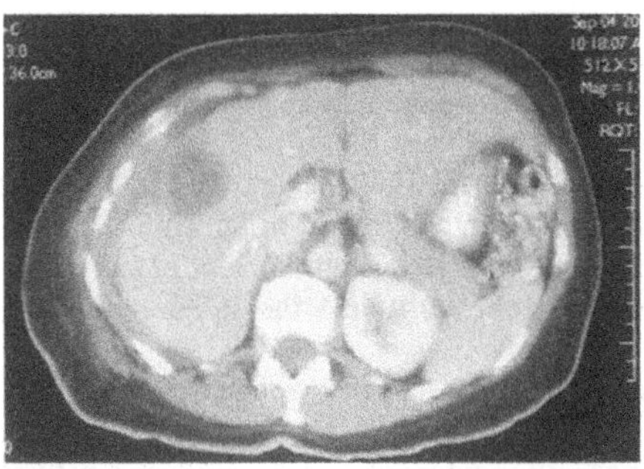

Fig. 7.23. CT scan: 66 year old lady with proven mesothelioma. There is an extensive tumour within the right hemithorax (not shown) which has directly invaded the liver having penetrated the diaphragm

References

Aberle D, Gamsu G, Ray C (1988) High-Resolution CT of Benign Asbestos-Related Diseases : Clinical and Radiographic Correlation. American Journal of Roentgenology 151:883-891

Aberle D, Gamsu G, Ray C, Feuerstein I (1988) Asbestos-related pleural and parenchymal fibrosis : detection with high-resolution CT. Radiology 166:729-734

Alexander E, Clark RA, Colley DB, Mitchell SE (1981) CT of malignant pleural mesothelioma. Am J Roentgenol 137: 287- 291

Al Jarad N, Poulakis N, Pearson M, Rubens M, Rudd R (1991) Assessment of asbestos-induced pleural disease by computed tomography - correlation with chest radiograph and lung function. Respiratory Medicine 85:203-208

Ameille J, Brochard P, Bréchot J, Pascano T, Cherin A, Raix A, et al. (1993) Pleural thickening: a comparison of oblique chest radiographs and high resolution computed tomography in subjects exposed to low levels of asbestos pollution. In: International Archives of Occupational and Environmental Health pp. 545-548

Baker E, Greene R (1982) Incremental value of oblique chest radiographs in the diagnosis of asbestos-induced pleural disease. American Journal of Industrial Medicine 3 (1):17-22

Bignon J (1989) Mineral fibres in the non occupational environment. In : Non occupational exposure to mineral fibres. In: Bignon J, Peto J, Saracci R (ed) IARC Scientific Publication n°90. Lyon. pp. 3-29

Boutin C, Dumortier P, Rey F, Viallat J, De Vuyst P (1996) Black spots concentrate oncogenic asbestos fibres in the parietal pleura. Thoracoscopic and mineralogic study. American Journal of Respiratory and Critical Care Medicine 153:444-449

Brenner J, Sordillo PP, Magill GB, Golbey RB(1982) Malignant mesothelioma of the pleura: Review of 123 patients. Cancer 49:2431-2439

Broderick A, Fuortes J, Merchant J, Galvin J, Schwartz D (1992) Pleural determinants of restrictive lung function and respiratory symptoms in an asbestos-exposed population. Chest 101:684 - 691

Churg A (1998) Nonneoplastic disease caused by asbestos. In: Churg A, Green F, (ed) Pathology of occupational lung disease. pp. 277-338

Copley S, Wells A, Rubens M, Chabat F, Sheehan R, Musk A, et al. (2001) Functional consequences of pleural disease evaluated with chest radiography and CT. Radiology 220(1):237-243

De Raeve H, Verschakelen J, Gevenois P, Mahieu P, Moens G, Nemery B (2001) Observer variation in computed tomography of pleural lesions in subjects exposed to indoor asbestos. European Respiratory Journal 17:916-921

De Vuyst P, Karjalainen A, Dumortier P, Pairon J, Monso E, Brochard P, et al. (1998) Guidelines for mineral fibre analyses in biological samples: report of the ERS Working Group. European Respiratory Society. European Respiratory Journal 11(6):1416-26

Edge JR, Choudhury SL (1978) Malignant mesothelioma of the pleura in Barrow-in-Furness. Thorax 33:26-30

Epler G, Fitzgerald M, Gaensler E, Carrington C (1980) Asbestos-related disease from household exposure. Respiration 39:229-240

Epler G, McLoud T, Gaensler E (1982) Prevalence and incidence of benign asbestos pleural effusion in a working population. Journal of American Medical Association 247:617 - 622

Fraser RS, Müller NL, Colman N, Paré PD(1999) Diagnosis of Disease of the chest 4th edition. WB Saunders, Philadelphia 4: Chapter 72

Friedman A, Fiel S, Fisher M, Radecki P, Lev-Toaff A, Df C (1988) Asbestos-related pleural disease and asbestosis : a comparison of CT and chest radiography. American Journal of Roentgenology 150:269-275

Ferguson DA, Berry G, Jelihovsky T, Andreas SB, Rogers AJ, Chung Fung S, Grimwood A, Thompson R (1987) The Australian Mesothelioma Surveillance Program 1979-1985. Med J Aust 147:166-172

Gevenois P, de Maertelaer V, Madani A, Winant C, Sergent G, De Vuyst P (1998) Asbestosis, pleural plaques and diffuse pleural thickening : three distinct benign responses to asbestos exposure. European Respiratory Journal 11:1021-1027

Gevenois P, Pichot E, Dargent F, Van De Weyer R, De Vuyst PAR (1994) Tomodensitométrie des pneumoconioses. Annales de Radiologie 37(3):222-228

Greenberg S (1992) Benign asbestos-related pleural disease. In: Roggli V, Greenberg S, Pratt P (ed) Pathology of asbestos-associated diseases. pp. 165-187

Greene R, Boggis C, Jantsch H (1984) Asbestos-related pleural thickening : effect of threshold criteria on interpretation. 152:569-573

Hillerdal G (1985) Nonmalignant pleural disease related to asbestos exposure. Clinical Chest Medicine 6:141-152

Hillerdal G (1989) Rounded atelectasis. Clinical experience with 74 patients. Chest 95:836-841

Hillerdal G, Özesmi M 1987) Benign asbestos pleural effusion : 73 exudates in 60 patients. European Journal of Respiratory Disease 71:113-121

Hiraoka T, Ohkura M, Morinaga K, Kohyama N, Shimazu K, Ando M (1998) Anthophyllite exposure and endemic pleural plaques in Kumamoto, Japan. Scandinavian Journal of Work Environment and Health 24(5):392-397

Im J, Webb W, Rosen A, Gamsu G (1989) Costal pleura : appearances at high-resolution CT. Radiology 171:125-131

International Labour Office (1980) International Labour Office guidelines for the use of the ILO international classification of radiographs of pneumoconiosis. Geneva

Jakobsson K, Stromberg V, Abin M, Welinder H, Hagman L (1995) Radiological changes in asbestos-cement workers. Occupational and Environmental Medicine 52:20-28

Kawashima A, Libshitz HI (1990) Malignant pleural mesothelioma: CT manifestations in 50 cases. Am J Roentgenol 155: 965-969

Koskinen K, Zitting A, Tossavainen A, Rinne J, Roto P, Kivekäs J, et al. (1998) Radiographic abnormalities among Finnish construction, shipyard and asbestos industry workers. Scandinavian Journal of Work Environment and Health 24:109-117

Lamphear BP, Buncher CR (1992) Latent period for malignant mesothelioma of occupational origin. J Occup Med 34: 718-721

Law MR, Gregor A, Husband JE, Kerr IH(1982) Computed tomography in the assessment of malignant mesothelioma of the pleura. Clin Radiol 33: 67-70

Lilis R, Lerman Y, Selikoff I (1988) Symptomatic benign pleural effusions among asbestos insulation workers: residual radiographic abnormalities. British Journal of Industrial Medicine 45:443-449

Lynch D, Gamsu G, Aberle D (1989) Conventional and high resolution computed tomography in the diagnosis of asbestos-related diseases. Radiographics 9:S23-S51

Lynch D, Gamsu G, Ray C, Aberle D (1988) Asbestos-related focal lung masses : manifestations on conventional and high-resolution CT scans. Radiology 169:603-607

Mc Hugh K, Blaquiere R (1989) CT features of rounded atelectasis. American Journal of Roentgenology 257-260

Mc Loud T, Woods B, Carrington C, Epler G, Gaensler E (1985) Diffuse pleural thickening in an asbestos-exposed population : prevalence and causes. American Journal of Radiology 144:9-18

Mirvis S, Dutcher JP, Haney PJ, Whitley NO, Aisner J (1983) CT of malignant pleural mesothelioma. Am J Roentgenol 140: 665-670

Müller NL (1993) Imaging of the pleura. Radiology 186: 297-309

Ohishi N, Oka T, Fukuhara T, Yotsumoto H, Yazaki Y (1996) Extensive pulmonary metastases in malignant pleural mesothelioma: A rare clinical and radiographic presentation. Chest 110: 296-298

Payne C, Jacques P, Ih K (1980) Lung folding simulating peripheral pulmonary neoplasm (Blesovsky's syndrome). Thorax 35:936-940

Peto J, Hodgson JT, Matthews FE, Jones JR (1995) Continuing increase in mesothelioma mortality in Britain. Lancet 345:535-539

Rockoff D, Kagan E, Schwartz A, Kriebel D, Hix W, Rohatgi P (1987) Visceral pleural thickening in asbestos exposure : the occurrence and implications of thickened interlobar fissure. Journal of Thoracic Imaging 2:58-66

Rogan W, Gladen B, Ragan N (1987) US prevalence of occupational pleural thickening : a look at chest X rays from the first national health and nutrition examination survey. American Journal of Epidemiology 126:893-900

Rosenstock L, Barnhart S, Heyer N, Pierson D, Hudson L (1988) The relationship among pulmonary function, chest roentgenographic abnormalities and smoking status in an asbestos-exposed cohort. American Review of Respiratory Disease 272-277

Rudd RM (1995) Asbestos-related disease. In: Brewis RAL, Corrin B, Geddes DM, Gibson GJ(ed) Respiratory Medicine 2nd edition. WB Saunders, Philadelphia 1:557-563

Sargent E, Gardanson J, Jacobson G, Bernbaum W, Shaut M (1978) Bilateral pleural thickening : a manifestation of asbestos dust exposure. American Journal of Roentgenology 131:579-585

Schwartz D (1991) New developments in asbestos-induced pleural disease. Chest 99:191-198

Schwartz D, Fuortes L, Galvin J, Burmeister L, Schmidt L, Leistikow B, et al. (1990) Asbestos-induced pleural fibrosis and impaired lung function. American Review of Respiratory Disease 141:321-326

Sider L, Holland E, Davis T, Cugell D (1987) Changes on radiographs of wives of workers exposed to asbestos. Radiology 164:723-726

Solomon A (1991) Radiological features of asbestos-related visceral pleural changes. American Journal of Industrial Medicine 19:339-355

Solomons K, Polakow R, Marchand P(1985) Diffuse malignant mesothelioma presenting as bilateral malignant lymphangitis. Thorax 40: 682-683

Teta MJ, Lewinsohn HC, Meigs JW, Vidone RA, Mowad LZ, Flannery JT (1983) Mesothelioma in Connecticut, 1955-1977: Occupational and geographic associations. J Occup Med 25:749-759

Van Cleemput J, De Raeve H, Verschakelen J, Rombouts J, Lacquet L, Nemery B (2001) Surface of localized pleural plaques quantitated by computed tomography scanning - No relation with cumulative asbestos exposure and no effect on lung function. American Journal of Respiratory and Critical Care Medicine 163(3):705-710

Wang X, Yano E, Wang M, Wang Z, Christiani D (2001) Pulmonary function in long-term asbestos workers in China. Journal of Occupational and Environmental Medicine 43 (7) 623-629

Webb W, Müller N, Naidich D (1996). High-resolution CT of the lung. Second edition ed. Philadelphia, New-York: Lippincott, Raven

Weiss W (1993) Asbestos-related pleural plaques and lung cancer. Chest 103:1854-1859.

Whitwell F, Rawcliffe RM (1971) Diffuse malignant pleural mesothelioma and asbestos exposure. Thorax 26: 6-22

Yates D, Browne K, Stidolph P, Neville E (1996) Asbestos-related bilateral diffuse pleural thickening : natural history of radiographic and lung function abnormalities. American Journal of Respiratory and Critical Care Medicine 153:301-306

Chapter 8 Parenchymal Changes of CT Imaging

Masanori Akira

Chief, Department of Radiology, National Kinki Central Hospital, 1180 Nagasone-cho, Sakai, Osaka 591-8025, Japan

Correlation with radiographic classification system

In the chest radiographic classification system associated with pneumoconiosis, the radiographic opacities are divided into two categories, small and large, with each defined in specific quantitative terms. An opacity of any size or shape that is larger than 10 mm in diameter is classified as a large opacity. With respect to small opacities, two shapes are recognized: small rounded and small irregular. According to the International Labour Office (ILO) 1980 International Classification of Radiographs of Pneumoconiosis, small rounded opacities smaller than 1.5 mm in diameter are classified as p; those between 1.5 and 3 mm, q; and those between 3 and 10 mm, r [1]. Opacities of the q and r types are characterized by sharply demarcated, rounded nodules or contracted nodules on HRCT (Fig. 8.1). In contrast, opacities of the p type are characterized by tiny branching lines or ill-defined punctate opacities, usually in a centrilobular location on HRCT (Fig. 8.2) [2]. Previous studies have shown that these tiny opacities correspond to irregular fibrosis around and along the respiratory bronchioles or dust macule with dilatation of respiratory bronchioles. In some patients with pneumoconiosis, nonperiperal, small areas of low attenuation with a central dot are found (Fig. 8.3). These small areas of low attenuation with a central dot have shown to correspond to focal dust emphysema. Focal emphysema has been most commonly founded in pneumoconiosis with p-type changes [2]. When small rounded opacities of the p type are few in number, that is profusion category 1, they are not easy to distinguish from pulmonary vessels. These opacities are similar to the appearance of pulmonary vessels because of their branching structure but differ in regional distribution; the opacities are intermingled with dots or minute, binary branching structures corresponding to pulmonary vessels, and there are many tiny opacities in part of a lobe compared with the surrounding, normal-appearing lung parenchyma [2].

HRCT appearances of small irregular opacities are various and include intralobular interstitial thickening, interlobular septal line, subpleural line, subpleural wedge-shaped nodular irregularity, parenchymal band, honeycombing, and ground-glass opacity.

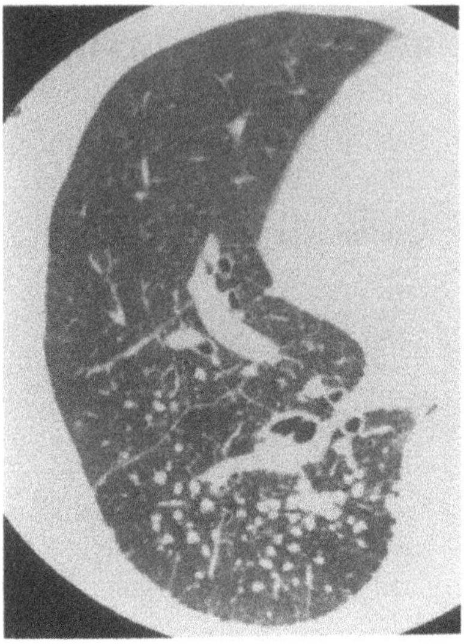

Fig. 8.1. HRCT scan of q type opacities. Opacities of predominant q type are seen. These nodules are sharply demarcated and rounded

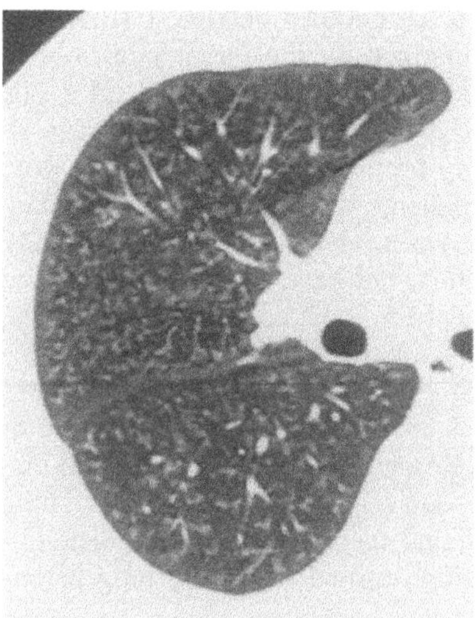

Fig. 8.2. HRCT scan of p type opacities. Numerous tiny branching lines of ill-defined punctate opacities, usually in a centrilobular location, are seen

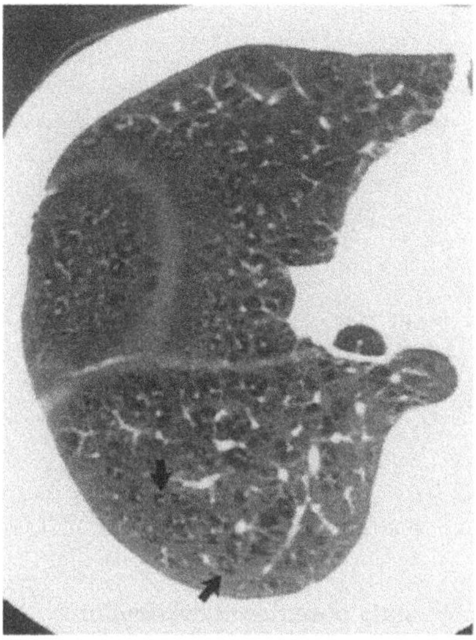

Fig. 8.3. HRCT scan of focal emphysema. Centrilobular areas of low attenuation with a central dot are seen (*arrows*)

CT imaging in silicosis

Silicosis is characterized by the presence of small discrete nodules extensively distributed in the upper zones of the lung, with a posterior predominance (Fig. 8.4). Micronodules can be detected in the subpleural areas, and confluence of the subpleural micronodules may simulate pleural plaques and is referred to as pseudoplaques (Fig. 8.5). Progressive massive fibrosis (PMF) is seen as irregularly shaped masses, most frequently in apical and posterior segments of upper and lower lobes, with peripheral parenchymal distortion (Fig. 8.6) [3]. Cavitation can occur from ischemic necrosis or accompanying tuberculosis. PMF and nodules may occasionally calcify. Low attenuation areas in PMF are sometimes seen. Cavitation usually occurs after large low attenuation area appears in PMF. As conglomeration develops, the affected lung loses volume and compensatory emphysema occurs in the unaffected portion.

Acute silicosis occurs in subjects exposed to very high concentrations of silica over periods of as little as a few weeks. The radiographic findings are similar to those in alveolar proteinosis. HRCT scans show a diffuse ground-glass or alveolar pattern.

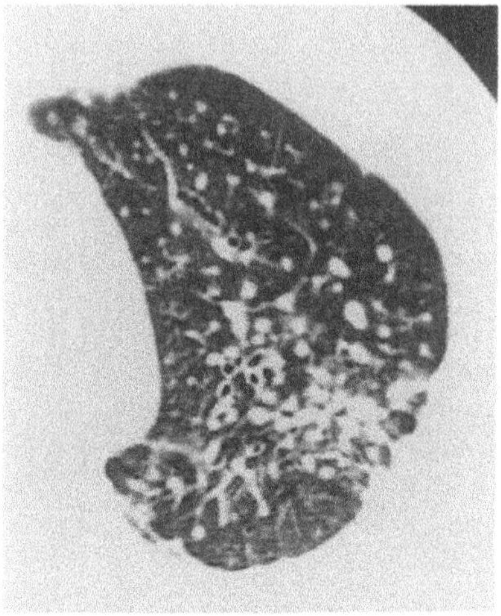

Fig. 8.4. HRCT scan of silicosis. Nodules are predominantly posterior in distribution

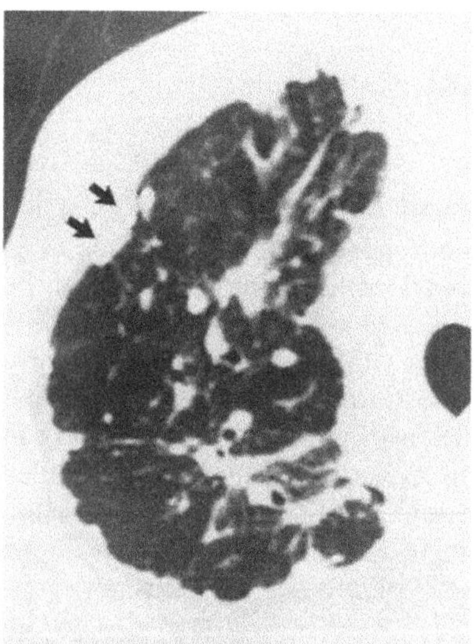

Fig. 8.5. HRCT scan of silicosis. Subpleural micronodules along the concavity of the chest wall mimic a pleural plaque (pseudoplaque) (*arrows*)

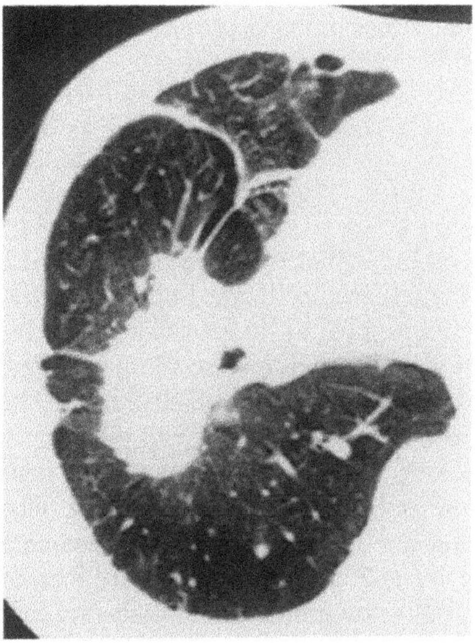

Fig. 8.6. HRCT scan of complicated silicosis. Progressive massive fibrosis (PMF) is seen in posterior segments of upper and lower lobes. Compensatory emphysema is seen around the PMF

CT imaging of coal worker's pneumoconiosis (CWP)

The inhalation of coal mine dust may lead to the development of coal worker's pneumoconiosis (CWP) and silicosis. The characteristic lesion of CWP is the collection of closely packed dust-laden macrophages around the respiratory bronchiole which contains little collagen, so-called coal dust manule. Another type of lesion is the fibrotic nodule. Reflected with the pathological findings, small nodular opacities are classified into two patterns: ill-defined tiny hyperattenuating areas that appear either as fine branching structures or as a few dots clustered together; or well-defined, discrete nodules. The appearance of PMF seen in CWP is similar to that in silicosis. However, histopathologically PMF of coal or other carbonaceous pneumoconiosis is distinguished from a silicotic conglomeration by the excess of black dust, and by the absence of individually identifiable silicotic nodules with their distinctive whorled pattern in the aggregate. Complicated pneumoconiosis is defined by the presence of nodules measuring 1 cm or more, that is PMF. Complicated pneumoconiosis is associated usually with a large amount of bullous scar emphysema. Central lesions tend to contact toward the hilum, whereas peripheral lesions are often seen with a thickening of overlying extrapleural fat [3].

Diffuse interstitial pulmonary fibrosis (DIPF) is sometimes found in the lungs of coal miners. The overall incidence of DIPF is approximately 18 percent [4]. DIPF in coal workers is associated with irregular opacities. Caplan's syndrome or rheumatoid pneumoconiosis consists of rounded discrete rheumatoid nodules ranging in size from 0.5 to 5 cm in diameter, superimposed on pneumoconiotic opacities. These nodules appear rapidly and often cavitate.

CT imaging of asbestosis

The common HRCT findings of asbestosis include thickened intralobular lines, irregular thickening of interlobular septae, subpleural curvilinear lines, parenchymal bands, ground-glass opacity, and honeycombing [5, 6]. In asbestosis, core regions of intralobular interstitium, that is centrilobular regions, are more affected. The thickened intralobular lines showed predominant subpleural distribution. The subpleural lesions appear as dotlike structures a few millimeters from the pleural surface. Some of them appear as fine branching structures, and some are connected with the most peripheral branch of the pulmonary artery (Fig. 8.7). The subpleural dotlike structures are arranged along the inner chest wall and resemble a curvilinear line (Fig. 8.8). Interlobular lines are 1–2 cm in length and are seen in the subpleural parenchyma, extending peripherally toward the pleural surface and contacting it. Subpleural curvilinear lines are defined as linear areas of increased attenuation seen within 1 cm of the pleura and parallel to the inner chest wall. Parenchymal bands are defined as linear densities from 2 to 5 cm in length coursing through the lung, usually to contact the pleura. Hazy patches of increased attenuation of various sizes are seen in the subpleural dependent or nondependent parenchyma, often accompanied by other architectural abnormalities. In the subpleural location, unlike gravity-dependent opacity, the hazy patches are discontinuously arranged and do not disappear when the patient is in the prone position. Small cystic spaces with thick walls are seen, mingled with other areas of increased attenuation. Honeycombing is defined as an accumulation of cystic spaces with thickened walls. Lobular areas of low attenuation, which represent areas of air-trapping, may be seen in the affected lung.

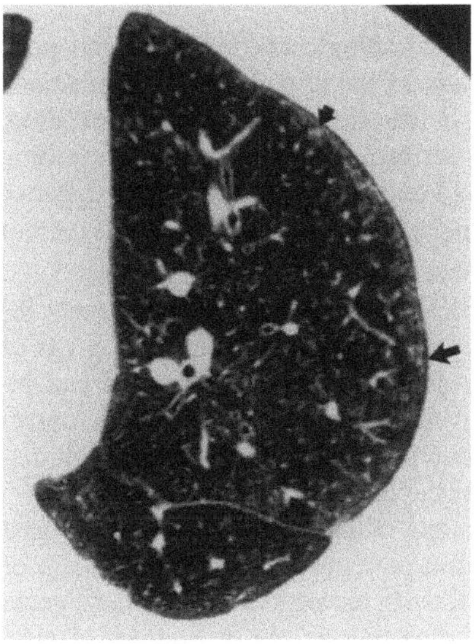

Fig. 8.7. HRCT scan of asbestosis. Thickened intralobular core lines. The subpleural lesions appear as dotlike structures a few millimeters from the pleural surface (*arrows*)

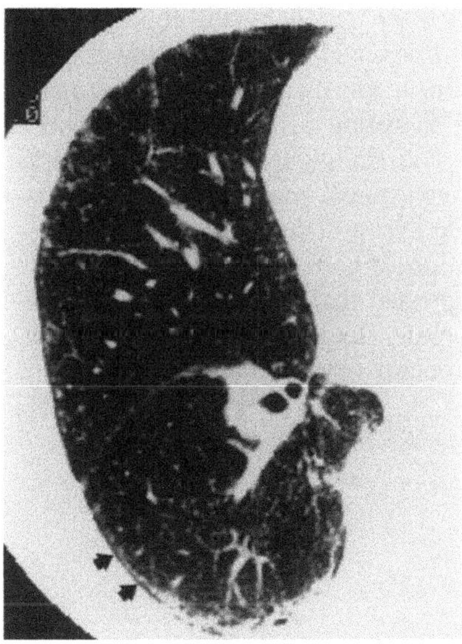

Fig. 8.8. HRCT scan of asbestosis. Subpleural dotlike lesions are arranged along the inner chest wall (*arrows*).

The thickened intralobular lines are shown histologically to be due to peribronchiolar fibrosis with subsequent involvement of the alveolar ducts. Thickened inlerlobular lines are due mainly to interlobular fibrotic or edematous thickening. Subpleural curvilinear lines correspond to peribronchiolar fibrotic thickening combined with flattening and collapse of the alveoli due to fibrosis. The distance of the subpleural curvilinear lines from the inner chest wall is never > 1.0 cm but is mostly < 0.5 cm [7]. The curvilinear lines observed at distance of about 1.5 – 2 cm from the inner chest wall are due to the thickened secondary lobular septa [8] or plate-like atelectasis in the corticomedullary junction of the lung [9]. Areas of ground-glass attenuation are shown to be the result of mild alveolar wall and interlobular septal thickening due to fibrosis or edema. Parenchymal bands correspond to fibrosis along the bronchovascular sheath or interlobular septa, with distortion of the parenchyma caused by traction of the thickened pleura [5].

To determine the earliest stage at which lesions in asbestosis can be diagnosed and to assess their progression, asbestos-exposed patients with profusion score of less than 1/1 were examined with serial HRCT, with an interval one – three years between examinations [10]. On the basis of the paired serial CT findings, Figure 8.9 shows progression of asbestosis on HRCT. The paired serial CT scans showed that subpleural isolated dots or branching lines connected with the most peripheral branch of the pulmonary artery stated to appear in lower subpleural zones and then became confluent to create pleural-based nodular irregularities and subpleural curvilinear lines. Ground-glass opacity appears around these parenchymal abnormalities. Later, small cystic spaces appear in these perenchymal abnormalities. Early findings in asbestosis include subpleural thickened intralobular lines, thickened interlobular septal lines, subpleural curvilinear lines, and ground-glass opacities, without lung distortion or with slight lung distortion. Honeycombing, traction bronchiectasis, and severe lung distortion are late findings of asbestosis. Parenchymal bands caused by traction of the thickened pleura may appear without asbestosis. Parenchymal bands are often associated with diffuse pleural thickening. Gevenois et al. [11] described that the association of parenchymal bands and diffuse pleural thickening in the same cluster suggested that these bands reflect visceral pleural fibrosis rather than interstitial fibrosis. Because of associated abnormalities of the pleura, " infolding " of the lung occurs (rounded atelectasis).

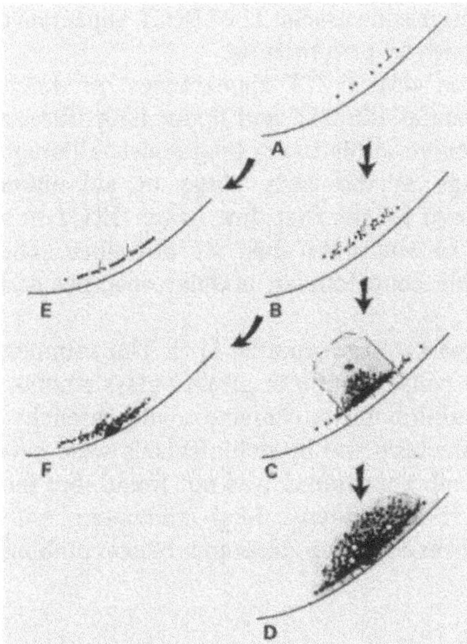

Fig. 8.9. Progression of asbestosis on HRCT. *A*; Dot-like lesions appear in the subpleural region. *B*; The dot-like lesions increase in number. *C*; Ground-glass opacity appears but with the lung architecture preserved. *D*; Small cystic spaces appear with lung distortion. *E*; The dot-like lesions create subpleural curvilinear lines. *F*; Pleural-based nodular opacities appear

CT imaging in other pneumoconioses

Four distinct forms of pulmonary disease caused by talc have been described. The first form, talcosilicosis, is caused by talc mined with high-silica-content mineral. Findings in this form are identical with those of silicosis. Talcoasbestosis closely resembles asbestosis and is produced by crystalline talc, generally inhaled with asbestos fibers. The third form, talcosis, caused by inhalation of pure talc, may include acute or chronic bronchitis as well as interstitial inflammation; radiographically, it appears as interstitial reticulations or small, irregular nodules, typical of small-airway obstruction (Fig. 8.10). The fourth form, due to intravenous administration of talc, is usually associated with abuse of oral medications and production of vascular granulomas manifested by consolidations, large nodules, and masses [12]

The typical HRCT findings in arc welder's siderosis are ill-defined micronodules diffusely distributed in the lung. Some of the micronodules appear as fine branching lines (Fig. 8.11). In less affected lung, micronodules show centrilobular distribution [13]. The micronodules do not reflect reactive fibrosis but, rather, radiopaque accumulations of iron particles that lie within macrophages, aggregated along the perivascular and peribronchial lymphatic vessels. The HRCT appearance sometimes resembles with that of hypersensitivity pneumonitis.

Aluminum pneumoconiosis can produce several CT appearances: predominantly reticular fibrosis; predominantly nodular fibrosis; and upper lung fibrosis [13] (Fig. 8.12). Fibrosis is usually most severe in the upper lung zones, although it may be diffused. The HRCT findings in the early stage of aluminum dust-induced changes that could be diagnosed for the first time using HRCT in a worker exposed long-term to high levels of aluminum dust are described. The HRCT findings were characterized by small, centrilobular, nodular opacities and slightly thickened interlobular septae [14].

The HRCT findings in two hard metal workers are reported [13]. The common HRCT findings included bilateral air space consolidation or ground-glass attenuation, which were mainly panlobular and multilobular in character, with parenchymal distortion (Fig. 8.13). Traction bronchiectasis and bronchiolectasis were evident in the consolidation. Typical honeycomb appearance was not found, but the presence of air bronchiolograms within areas of intense lung attenuation with parenchymal distortion suggested the existence of microscopic honeycombing [13].

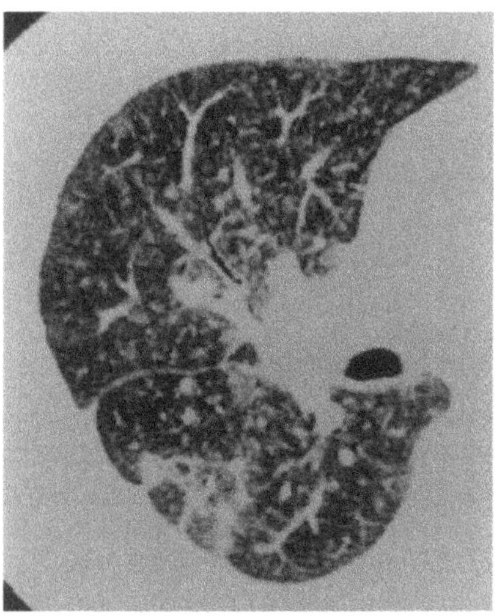

Fig. 8.10. HRCT scan of talcosis. Diffusely distributed ill-defined small nodules and ground-glass opacity are seen

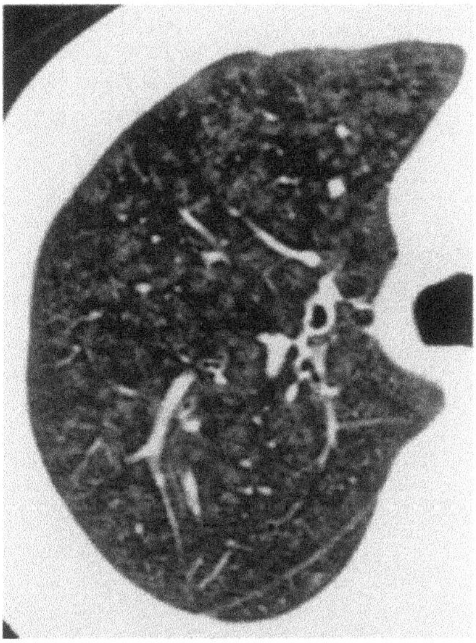

Fig. 8.11. HRCT scan of siderosis. Ill-defined centrilobular nodular areas of ground-glass attenuation diffusely distribute throughout the lung. The HRCT appearance resembles that of hypersensitivity pneumonitis

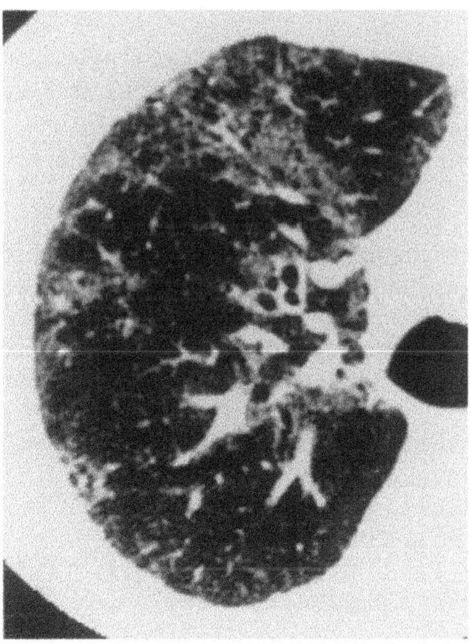

Fig. 8.12. HRCT scan of aluminum pneumoconiosis. Areas of ground-glass attenuation with intralobular interstitial thickening and traction bronchiectasis is seen

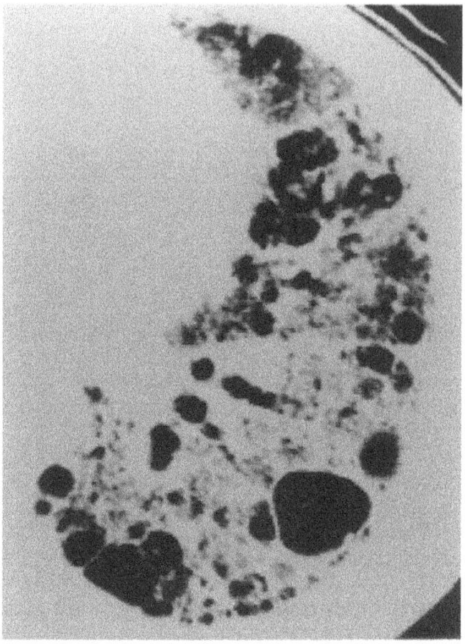

Fig. 8.13. HRCT scan of hard metal pneumoconiosis. Multilobular consolidation with bullae and traction bronchiectasis and bronchiolectasis is seen

References

International Labour Office: Guidelines for the use of ILO international classification of radiographs of pneumoconiosis, revised ed. International Labour Office Occupational Safety and Health Series N° 22 (rev 80). Geneva, International Labour Office, 1980

Akira M, Higashihara T, Yokoyama K, Yamamoto S, Kita N, Morimoto S, Ikezoe J, Kozuka T. Radiographic type p pneumoconiosis: thin-section CT. Radiology 1989; 171: 117-123

Remy-Jardin M, Remy J, Farre I, Marquette CH. Computed tomographic evaluation of silicosis and coal worker's pneumoconiosisd. Radiologic Clinics of North America 1992; 30: 1155-1175

Green FHY. Coal workers' pneumoconiosis and pneumoconiosis due to other carbonaceous dusts. In Churg A, Green FHY (eds): Pathology of Occupational Lung Disease. New York, Igaku-Shoin, 1988, 89-154

Aberle DR, Gamsu G, Ray CS, Feuerstein IM. Asbestos-related pleural and parenchymal fibrosis: detection with thin-section CT. Radiology 1988; 166: 729-734

Akira M, Yamamoto S, Yokoyama K, Kita N, Morinaga K, Higashihara T, Kozuka T. Asbestosis: thin-section CT-pathologic correlation. Radiology 1990; 176: 389-394

Yoshimura H, Hatakeyama M, Otsuji H, Maeda M, Ohishi H, Uchida H, Kasuga H, Katada H, Narita N, Mikami R, Konishi Y. Pulmonary asbestosis: CT study of curvilinear shadow. Radiology 1986; 158: 653-658

Naidich DP, Zerhouni EA, Siegelman SS: Computed tomography of the thorax. New York: Raven, 1984, 201

Kubota H, Hosoya T, Kato M, Uchimura F, Itagaki T, Yamaguchi K. Plate-like atelectasis at thew corticomedullary junction of the lung; CT observation and hypothesis. Radiat Med 1983; 1: 305-310

Akira M, Yokoyama K, Yamamoto S, Higashihara T, Morinaga K, Kita N, Morimoto S, Ikezoe J, Kozuka T. Early asbestosis: evaluation with thin-section CT. Radiology 1990; 178: 409-416

Gevenois PA, de Maertelaer V, Madani A, Winant C, Sergent G, De Vuyst P. Asbestosis, pleural plaques and diffuse pleural thickening: three distinct benign responses to asbestos exposure. Eur Respir J 1998; 11: 1021-1027

Feigin DS. Talc: understanding its manifestations in the chest. AJR 1986; 146: 295 – 301.

Akira M. Uncommon pneumoconioses: CT and pathologic findings. Radiology 1995; 197: 403-409

Kraus T, Schaller KH, Angerer J, Letzel S. Aluminum dust-induced lung disease in the pyro-powder-producing industry: detection by high-resolution computed tomography. Int Arch Occup Environ Health 2000; 73: 61-64

Chapter 9 Radiological and Pathological Correlation of Autopsied Cases of Pneumoconioses

Hiroaki Arakawa[1], Hisao Shida[2], Koichi Honma[3], and Yutaka Hosoda[4]

[1]Department of Radiology, Dokkyo University School of Medicine, Japan

[2]Department of Radiology, Rosai Hospital for Silicosis, Japan

[3]Department of Pathology, Dokkyo University School of Medicine, Japan

[4]Institute of Radiation Effects, Japan

In this chapter, we provide case presentations of various pneumoconioses with radiological and pathologic correlation. Included here are classical silicosis, asbestosis, talcosis, arc-welder's pneumoconiosis and mixed dust pneumoconiosis. In recent years, the incidence of classical silicosis is on the decline, whereas mixed dust pneumoconiosis has become increasingly frequent and, thereafter, has got the importance in clinical setting. A few years ago, based on this recognition, the authors held an international meeting about mixed dust pneumoconiosis and made clear its clinical and pathologic findings and proposed its definition (1). We briefly describe the concept and definition of mixed dust pneumoconiosis.

Definition of mixed dust pneumoconiosis (MDP)

Mixed dust here does not mean mixed dusts of any kind. A consensus was reached in terms of the definition of mixed dust pneumoconiosis at the Nikko Symposium in 1997 (1)—

1) Mixed dust pneumoconiosis (MDP) is caused by occupational exposure to crystalline silica (less than 18%) and non-fibrous silicates including talc, mica, and kaolinite.
2) Pathologically, MDP is defined as a pneumoconiosis composed of a combination of dust macules and mixed dust fibrosis with or without a small number of silicotic nodules or massive fibrosis.
3) Jobs probably causing mixed dust pneumoconiosis include foundry, welding, stone processing, production and handling of diatomite and concrete, cosmetics (containing talc or diatomite), construction of tunnels and dams, gravel collection, and building demolition.

Manifestation of MDP in relation to dust exposure level in workplace

The growing incidence of MDP is closely related to the improvement of dust exposure level so far (2).

In Japan, the governmental regulation of dust exposure level in ore mining began at 1948, when dramatic change in ore mining method ensued (3).

In the high exposure period (before 1950), the predominant type of disease was silicosis. Many of the patients had large opacities in addition to small rounded opacities, and showed severe impairment in their respiratory physiology. About 30% were complicated with tuberculosis, which did not respond to the therapeutic regimen at that time (2). Most of them died within 3 years after hospitalization.

In the low-level exposure period (after 1950), the disease had gradually shifted toward MDP with a decreased profusion of small rounded opacities and an increased prevalence of irregular opacities. Patients have become to live longer but at the same time the incidence of lung cancer increased in the elderly pneumoconiotics. In recent years (1970-) when exposure level has become minimal, not only the profusion of small rounded opacity but also the incidence of pneumoconiosis has dramatically been reduced.

All the cases presented here are selected from a large series of pneumoconiotics treated and autopsied in Rosai Hospital for Silicosis for the past 50 years (4). We believe that these cases provide important and useful information about pneumoconiosis that occurred in Japan in the last century.

Case 1

A case of mixed dust pneumoconiosis in a 77-year-old man who worked as a hauler in a metal mine for 24 years. Died of double lung cancers. He has been a life-long smoker.

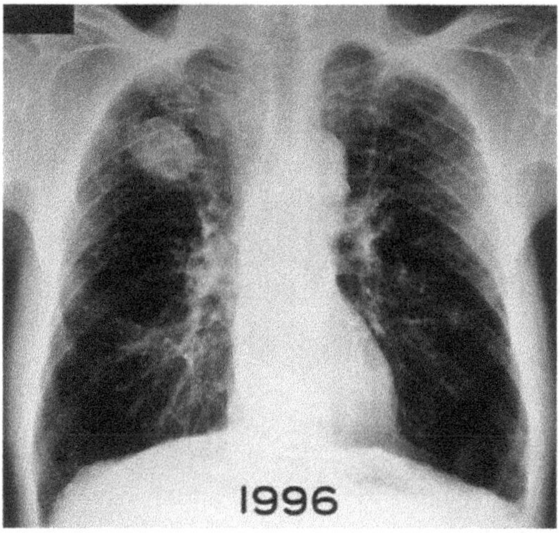

Fig. 9.1. A PA chest radiograph reveals a few numbers of small rounded opacities and irregular opacities in both upper lung zones. A well-defined mass, 4 cm in diameter, is noted in the right upper lobe. Pulmonary vessels have become sparse and overinflation of the lung is obviously identified. The radiograph is read as 1/1, p/s with symbol ca according to ILO classification

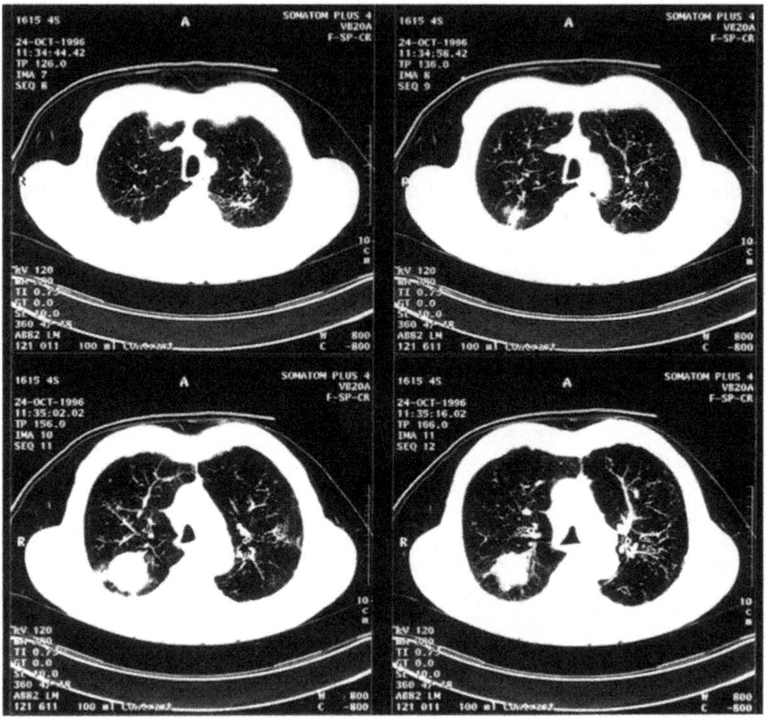

Fig. 9.2. CT scans demonstrate a round mass in the right upper lobe with lobulated contour, suggesting a probable lung cancer. Obvious pulmonary emphysema and small nodular opacities are noted as well

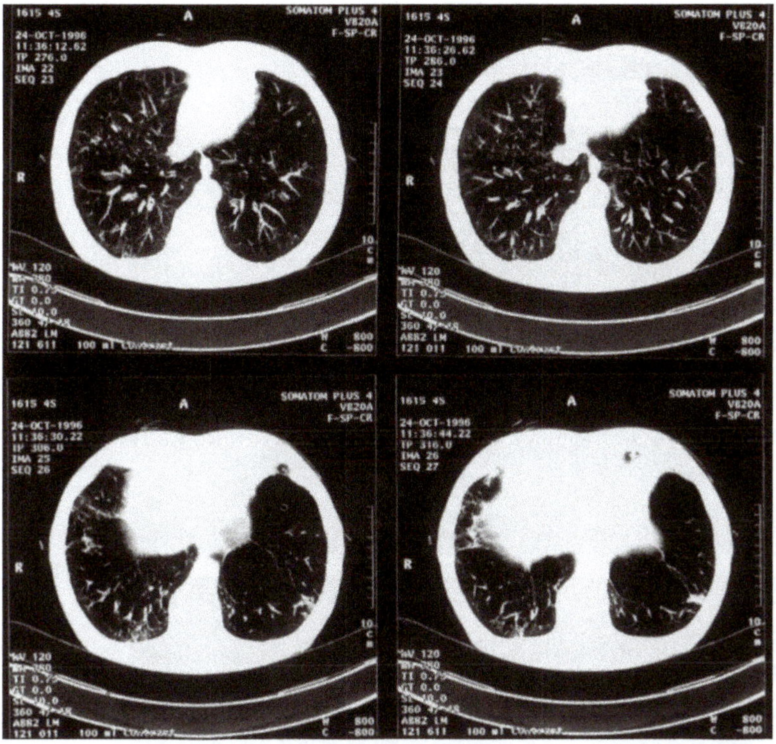

Fig. 9.3. CT scans at the lower levels show advanced pulmonary emphysema

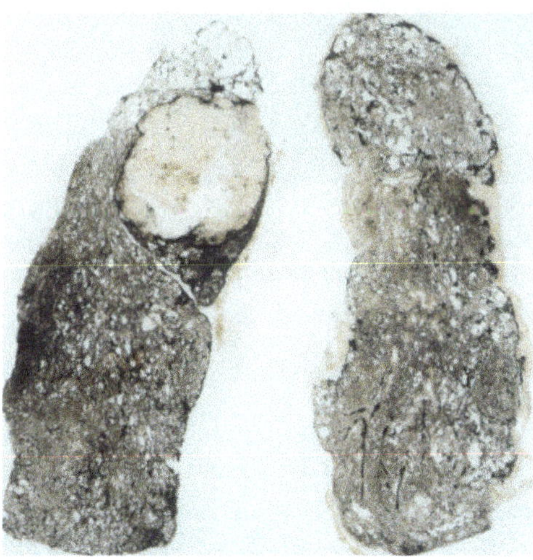

Fig. 9.4. Gough-Wentworth whole lung section demonstrates large tumor replacing the right upper lobe, sparse pigmented fibrous nodules and advanced emphysematous change

Histological findings—

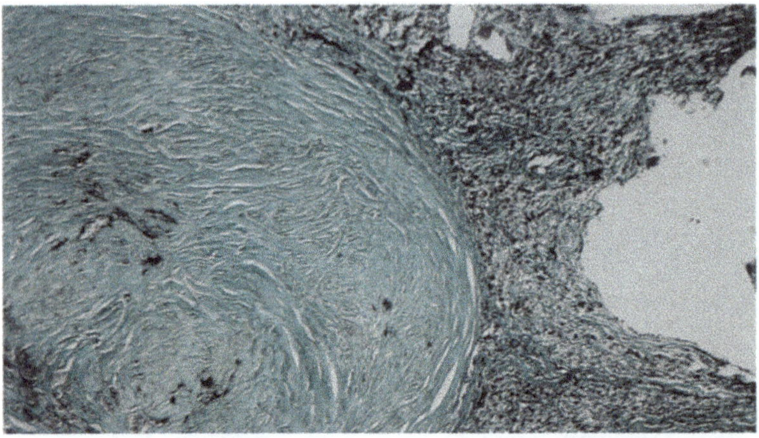

a

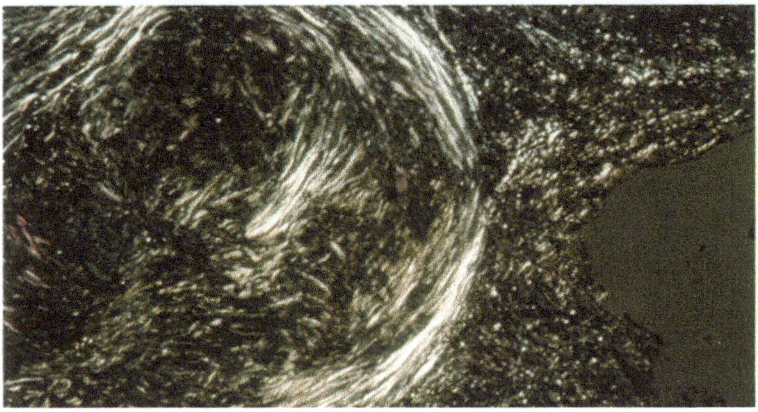

b

Fig. 9.5a, b. Magnified image of silicotic nodule by Elastica-Goldner stain (a). Under polarized light (b), sparse birefringent dust particles (silicate) are identified

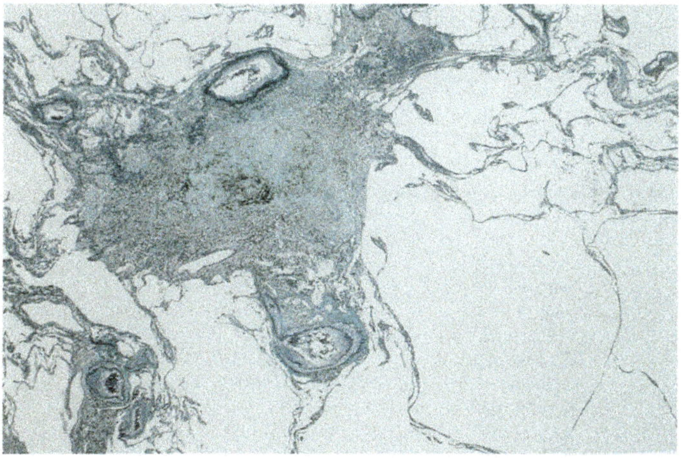

Fig. 9.6. Mixed dust fibrosis with marked emphysema

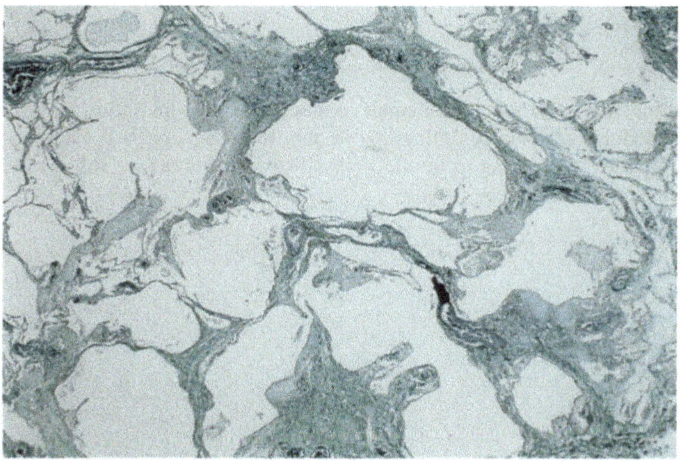

Fig. 9.7. Diffuse interstitial fibrosis with microscopic honeycombing

Case 2

A case of classical silicosis.
A 67-year-old man who worked in coal mines as a driller for 13 years. Died of congestive heart failure.

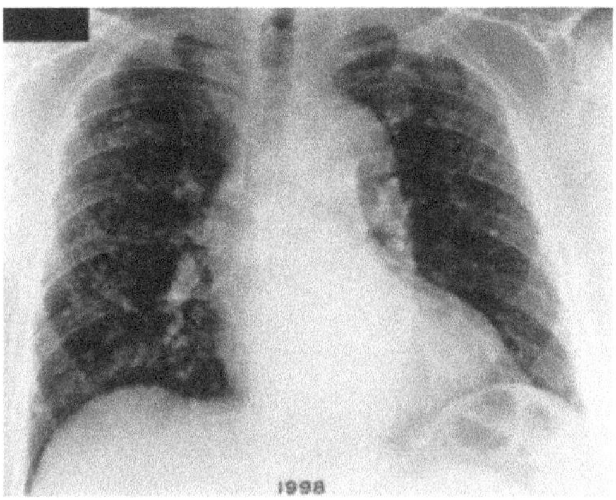

Fig. 9.8. A PA chest radiograph reveals multiple small rounded opacities involving all lung zones bilaterally. These nodules are clearly defined. Note that there are eggshell calcifications in both hilar lymph nodes. According to the ILO classification, this radiograph is read as 2/2 q/q and es

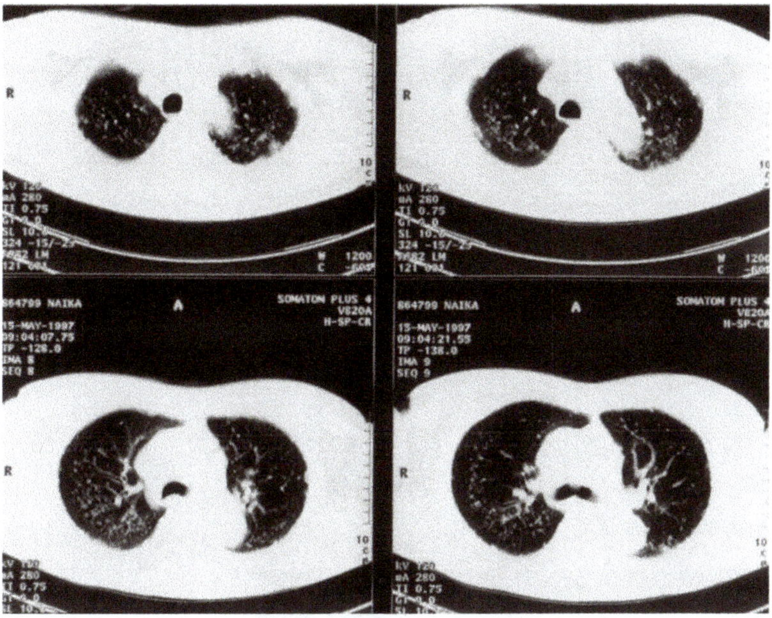

Fig. 9.9. Spiral CT scans obtained with 10-mm collimation demonstrate well-defined nodules in all lung zones with slight predominance in the upper lobes

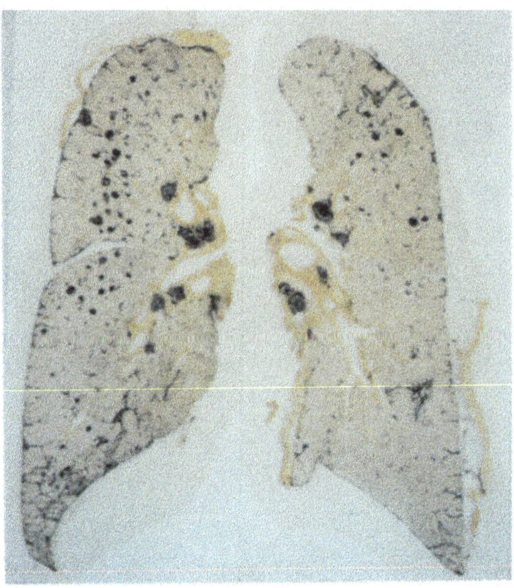

Fig. 9.10. Gough-Wentworth whole lung section demonstrates scattered silicotic nodules throughout the lungs and heavy deposition of dust in the hilar lymph nodes

Histological findings—

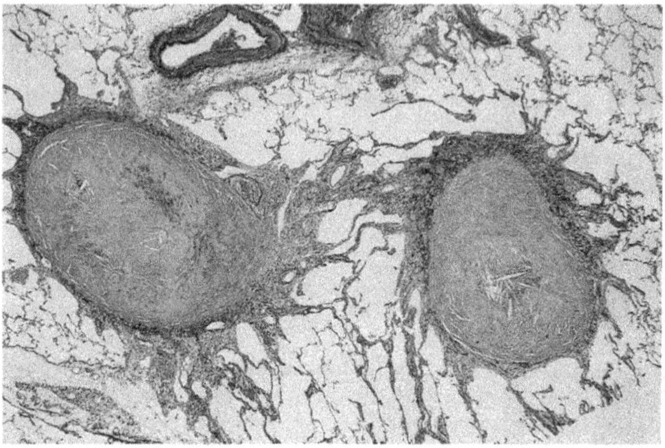

Fig. 9.11. Silicotic nodules

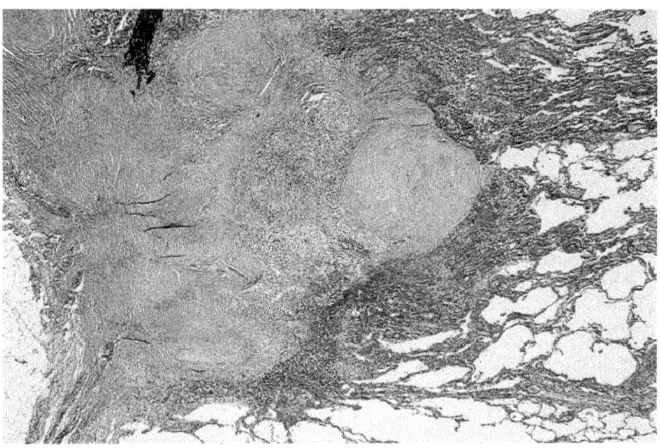

Fig. 9.12. Confluent nodules in the subpleural parenchyma that is associated with fibrous pleural adhesion

Case 3

A case of mixed dust pneumoconiosis and lung cancer.
An 86-year-old man who worked as a hauler in a metal mines for 24 years and died of lung cancer.

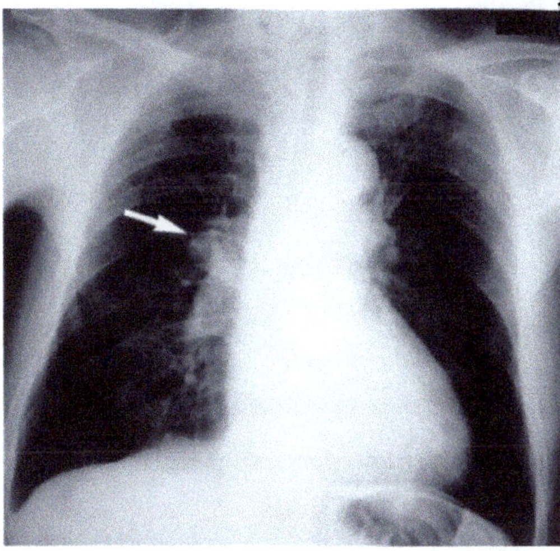

Fig. 9.13. A PA chest radiograph reveals a small number of q-size small rounded opacities in both upper lung zones. A larger nodule is noted in the right hilar area (*white arrow*).The ILO classification is 1/1 q/q, ca

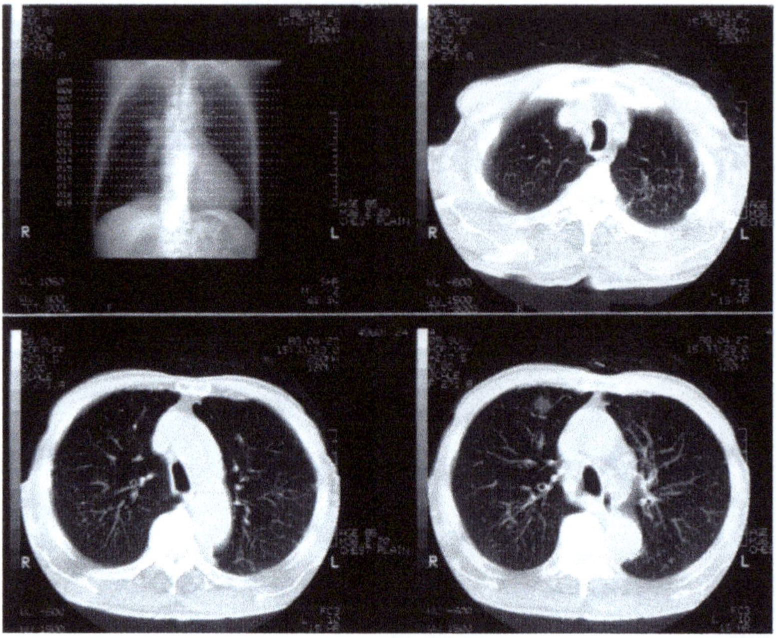

Fig. 9.14. CT scans with 10-mm collimation at upper lung zones show multiple tiny nodules in the posterior portion of both upper lobes

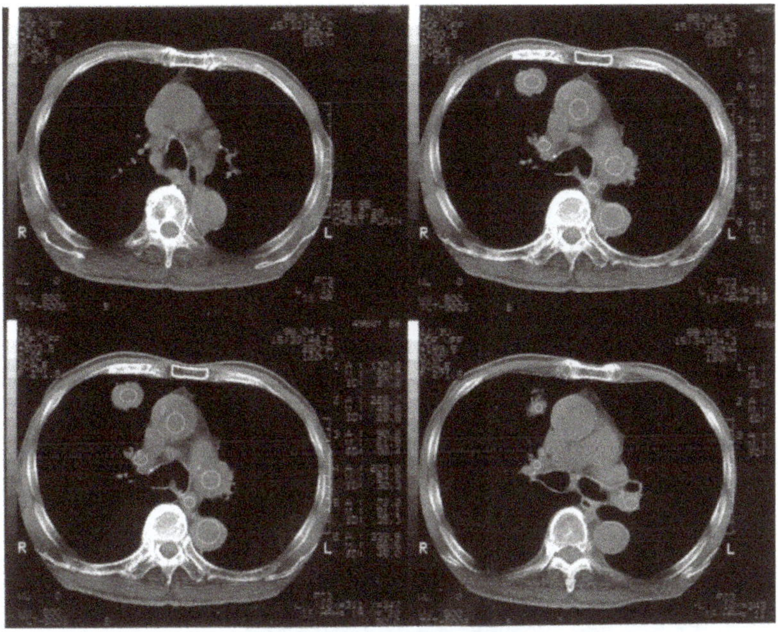

Fig. 9.15. CT scans with mediastinal window setting shows a nodule of 2-cm in diameter in the periphery of right upper lobe

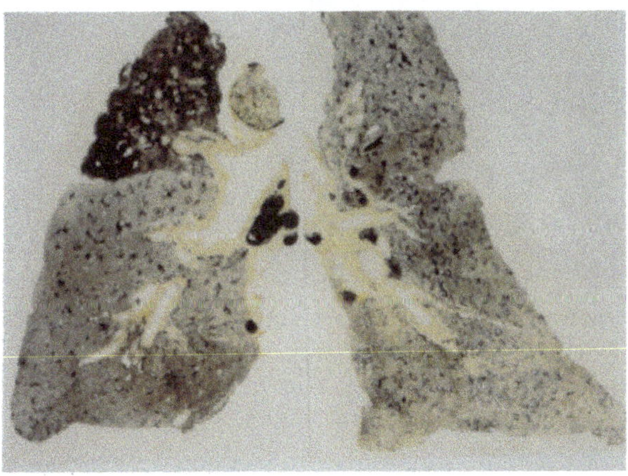

Fig. 9.16. Gough-Wentworth whole lung section shows moderate number of pigmented fibrous nodules, collapsed right upper lobe and pigmented hilar lymph nodes

Histologic findings –

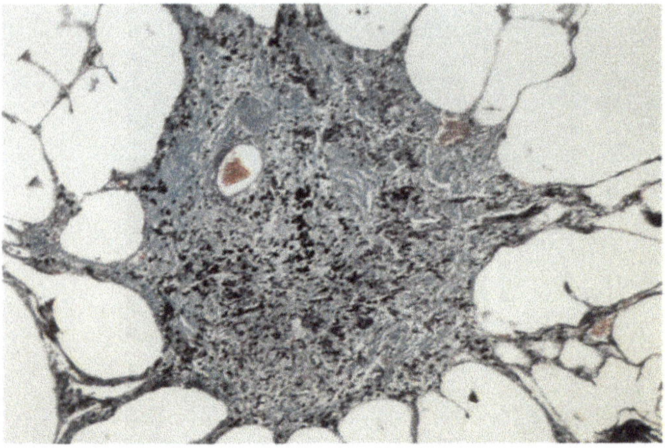

a

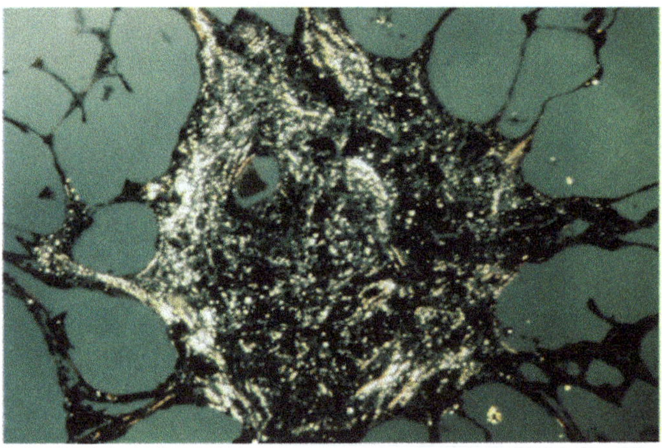

b

Fig. 9.17a, b. Mixed dust fibrosis shown for stellate nodules with birefringent dust particles deposited in the nodule (b; under polarized light)

Case 4

A case of mixed dust fibrosis and diffuse interstitial fibrosis.
An 85-year-old man who was a pit worker in a metal mine for 33 years. He died of lung cancer (small cell carcinoma).

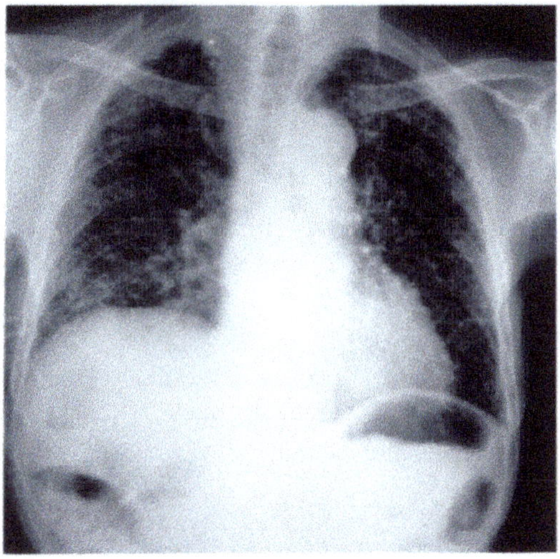

Fig. 9.18. A PA chest radiograph reveals densely distributed irregular opacities throughout the lungs with honeycombing. Elevation of the right hemi-diaphragm is noted. The ILO classification is 2/2 s/s, ho

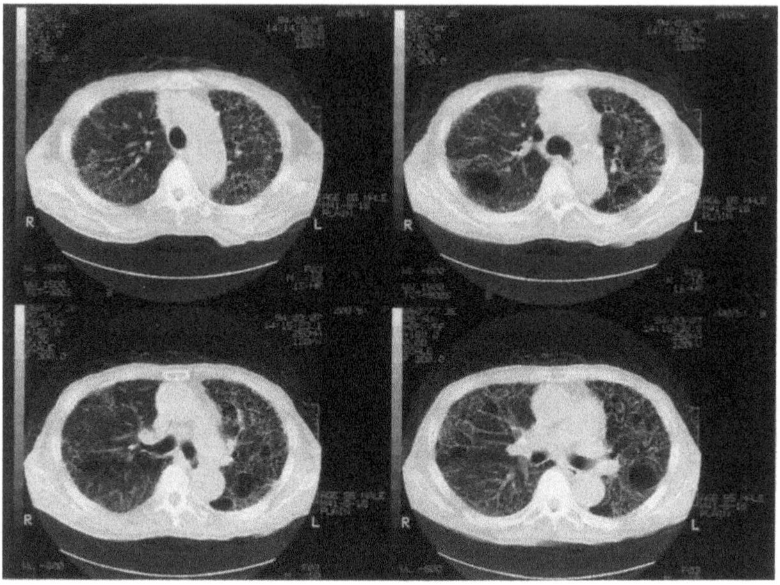

Fig. 9.19. CT images of the upper and middle lung zones demonstrate diffuse interstitial fibrosis with honeycombing. There are multiple large bullae as well

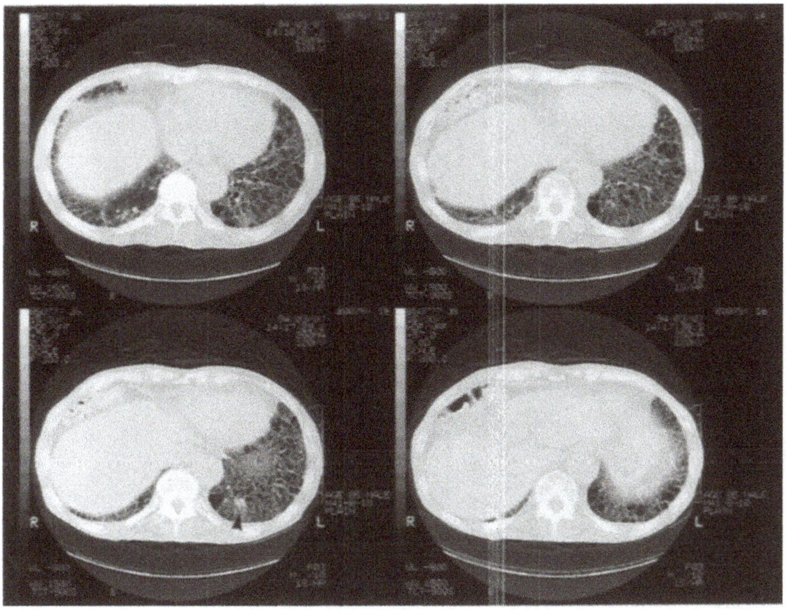

Fig. 9.20. CT images of the lower lung zones show extensive areas of honeycombing and an irregular shaped nodule in the left lower lung posteriorly (*arrowhead*), suggesting a possible lung cancer

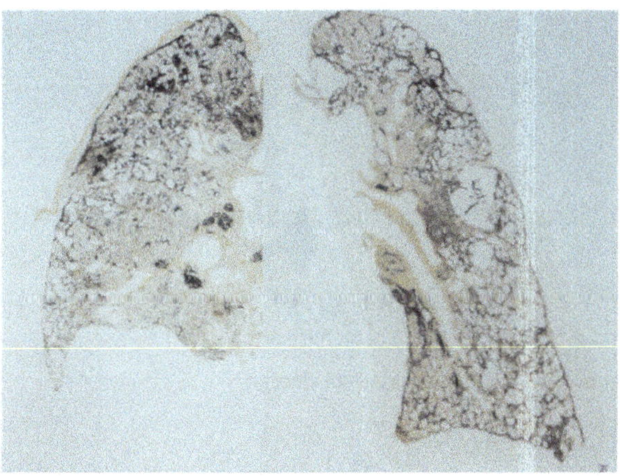

Fig. 9.21. Gough-Wentworth whole lung section demonstrates diffuse interstitial fibrosis in the lower lobes and sporadic pigmented fibrous nodules in the upper lobes

Histologic findings—

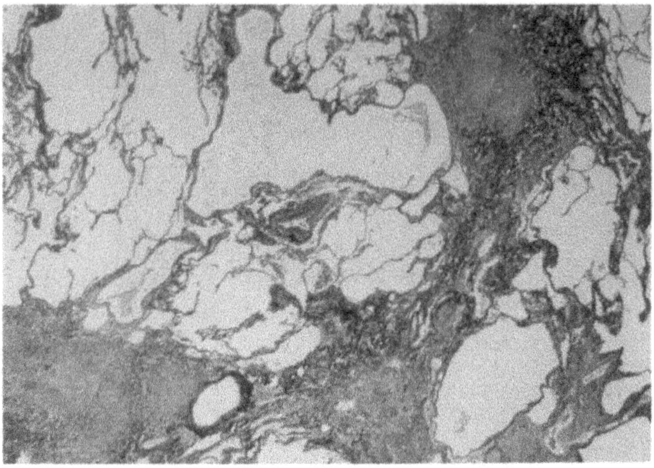

Fig. 9.22. Advanced diffuse interstitial fibrosis with honeycombing

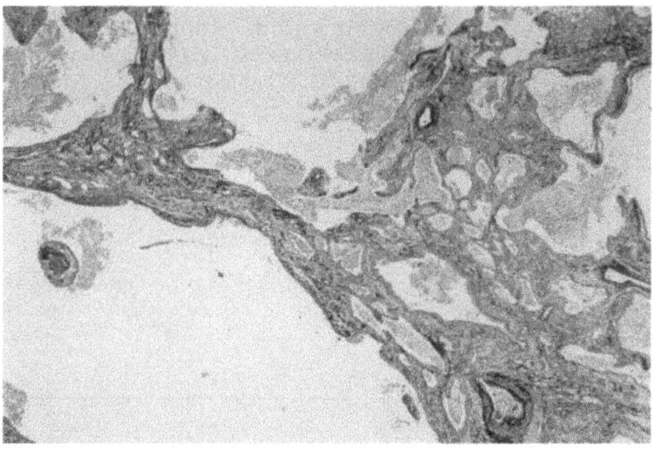

Fig. 9.23. Mixed dust fibrotic nodules with emphysematous change

Case 5

A case of mixed dust pneumoconiosis in a 71-year-old man who worked in a foundry as an arc welder for 30 years. He died of respiratory failure.

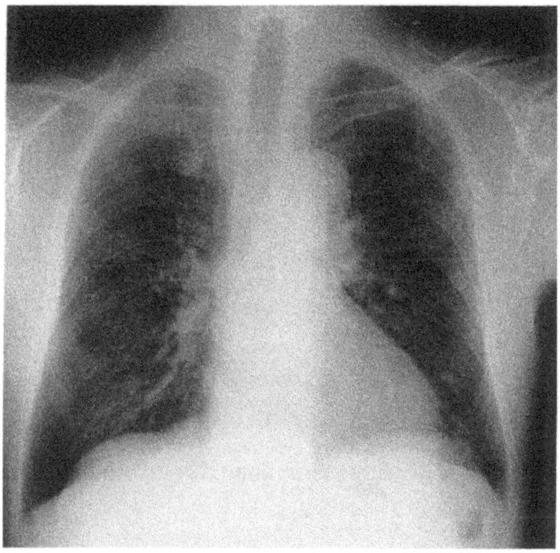

Fig. 9.24. A PA chest radiograph reveals densely scattered tiny rounded opacities throughout the lungs. The ILO classification is 2/2, p/p

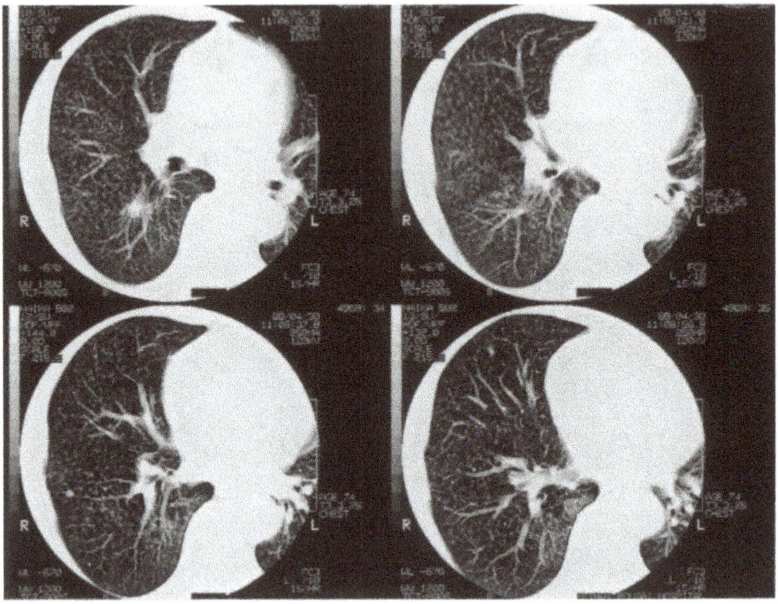

Fig. 9.25. Magnified CT images of right lung show densely disseminated small nodules that are located centrilobularly

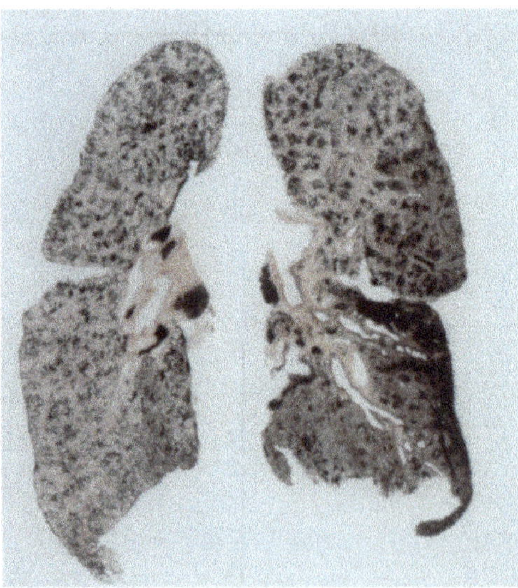

Fig. 9.26. Gough-Wentworth whole lung section shows sporadic pigmented fibrous nodules, dust macules and centrilobular emphysema

Histologic findings—

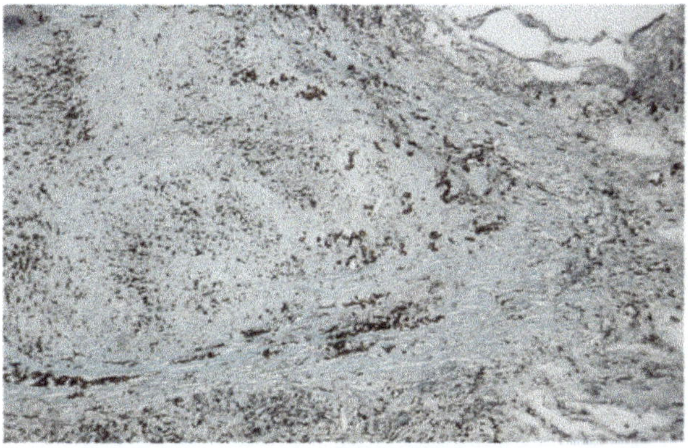

a

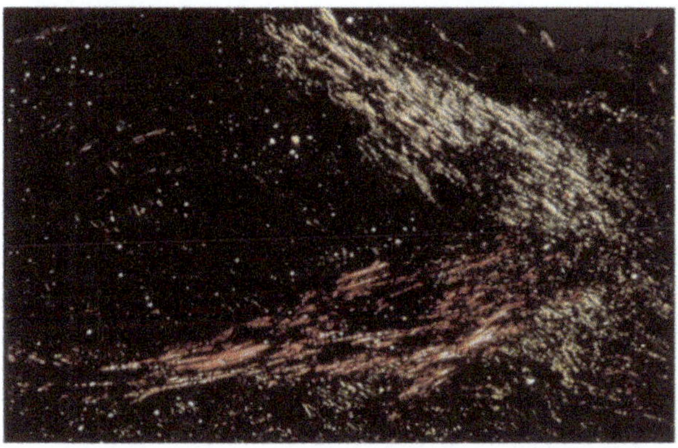

b

Fig. 9.27a, b. A degenerated silicotic nodule with birefringent dust particles under polarized light

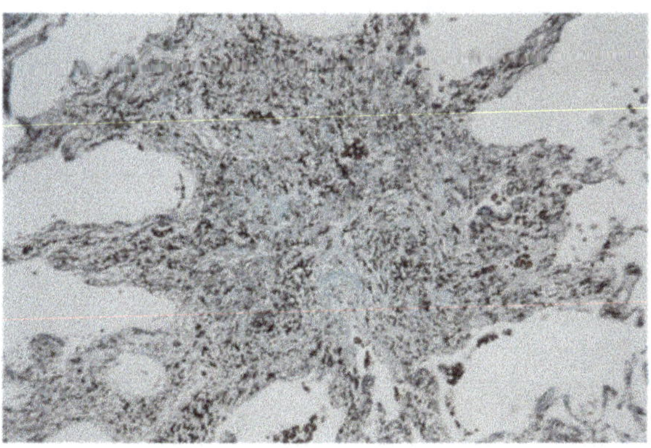

Fig. 9.28. A stellate nodule of mixed dust fibrosis with deposition of birefringent dust particles

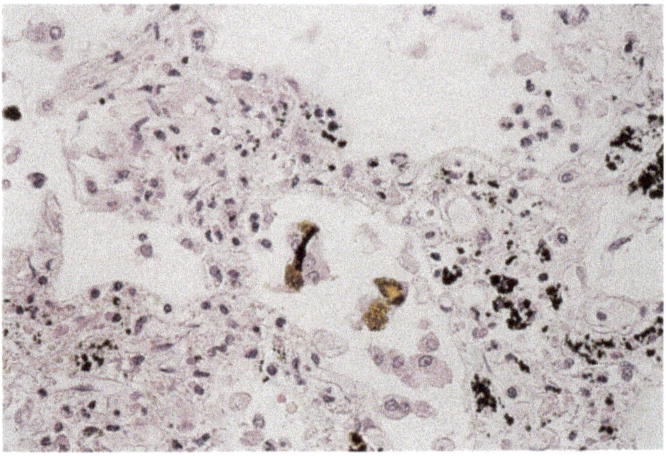

Fig. 9.29. Non-asbestos ferruginous body showing a black fibrous core

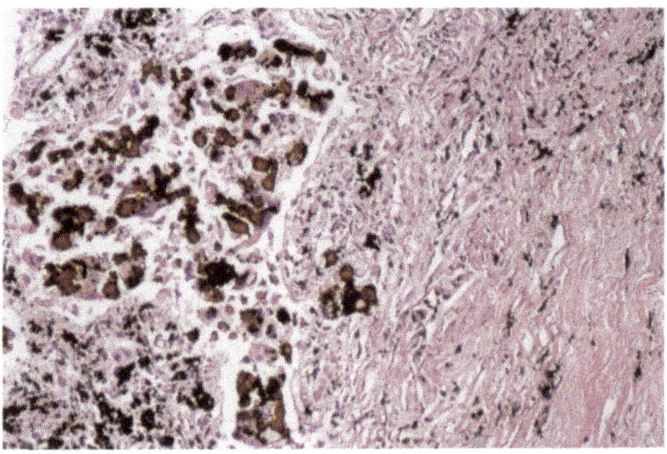

Fig. 9.30. A cluster of ferruginous bodies adjoining the fibrotic area

Case 6

A case of asbestosis in an 84-year-old man who worked in a foundry for 42 years. He died of lung cancer.

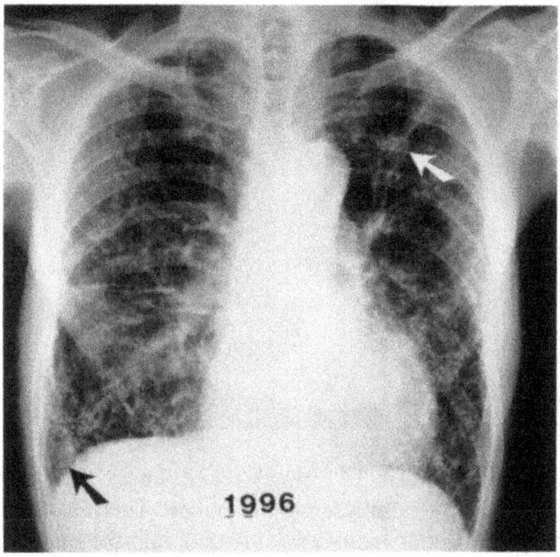

Fig. 9.31. A PA chest radiograph reveals diffuse irregular opacities of s-size throughout both lungs. There are two small irregular tumours in the right costophrenic angle (*black arrow*) and in the left upper lobe (*white arrow*), respectively. The appearance suggests lung cancers. The ILO classification is 3/3, s/s, ca, pi, ho, pc

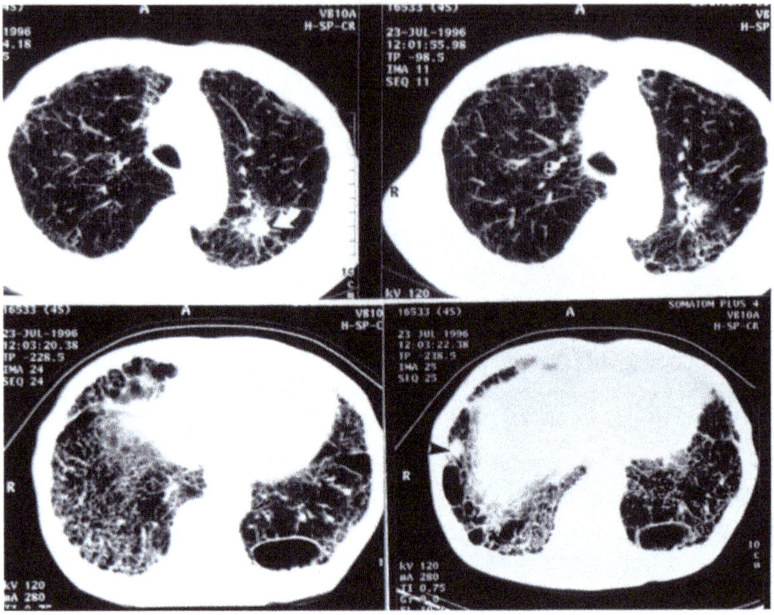

Fig. 9.32. CT images demonstrate dense distribution of reticular and linear opacities throughout the lungs accompanied with pulmonary emphysema and bullae. There are two nodules suggesting lung cancers, one in the left upper lung (*white arrow*), and the other in the right lower lung (*black arrowheads*)

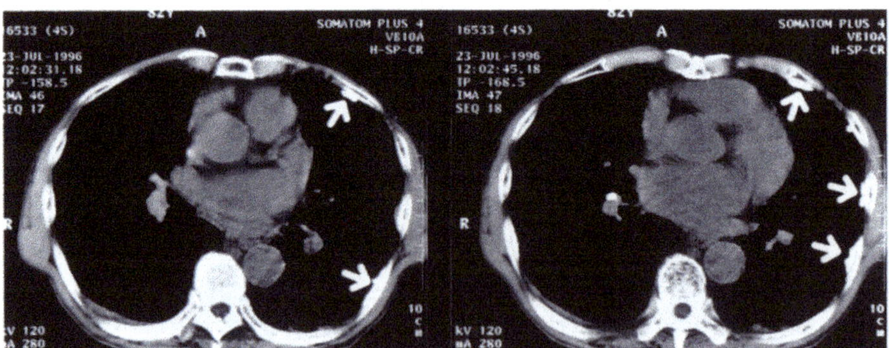

Fig. 9.33. CT images with mediastinal window setting show calcified plaques in the left middle lung zones, suggesting asbestos-related pleural abnormalities (*white arrows*)

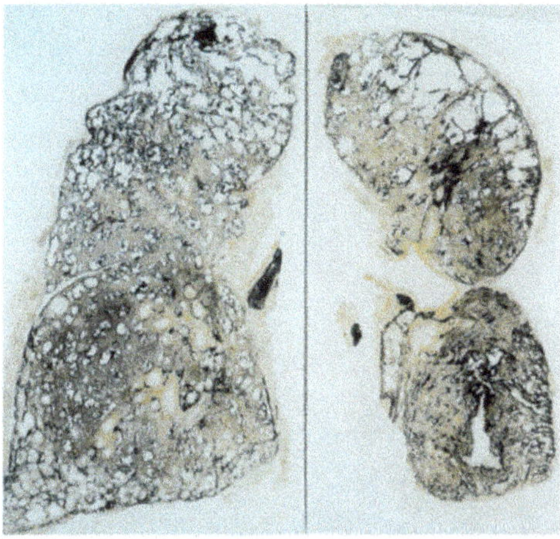

Fig. 9.34. Gough-Wentworth whole lung sections reveal diffuse interstitial fibrosis, sporadic pigmented nodules and markedly emphysematous parenchyma

Histologic findings—

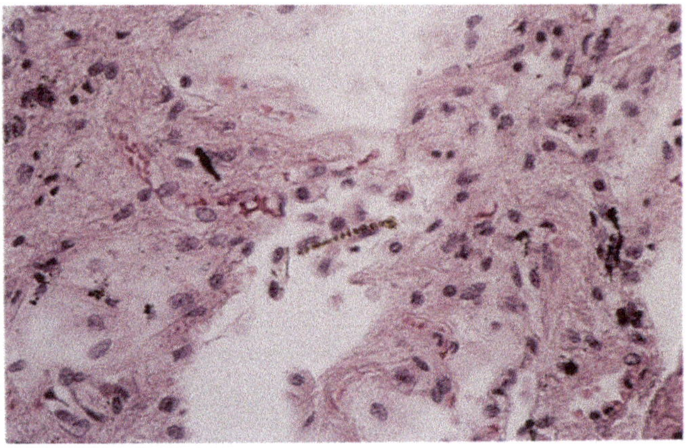

Fig. 9.35. Intra-alveolar asbestos body

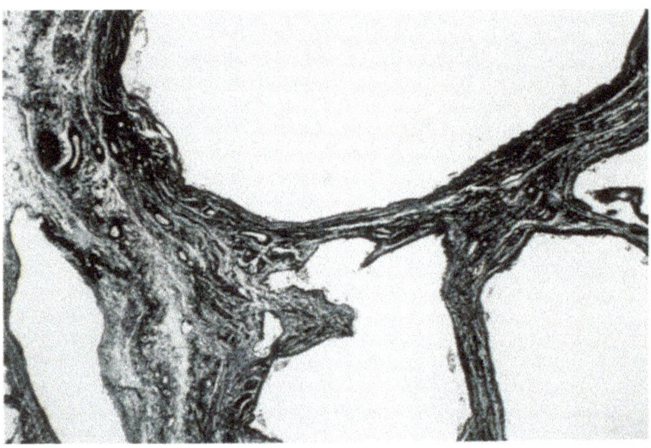

Fig. 9.36. Diffuse interstitial fibrosis with honeycombing

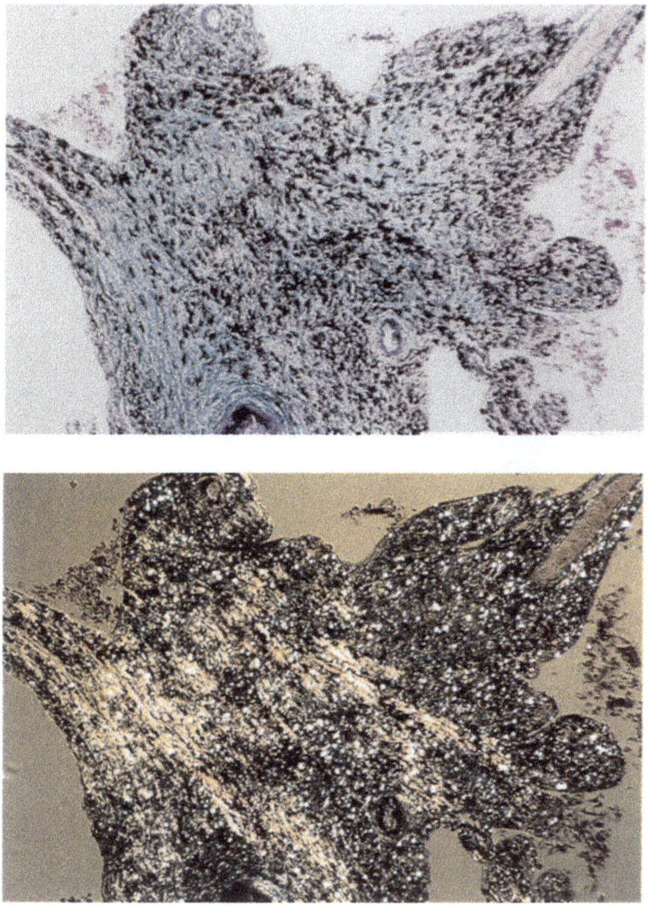

a

b

Fig. 9.37a, b. Mixed dust fibrosis having a large amount of birefringent dust particles under polarized right

Case 7

A case of asbestosis associated in a 59-year-old man.
He engaged in asbestos spraying for 22 years and died of respiratory failure.

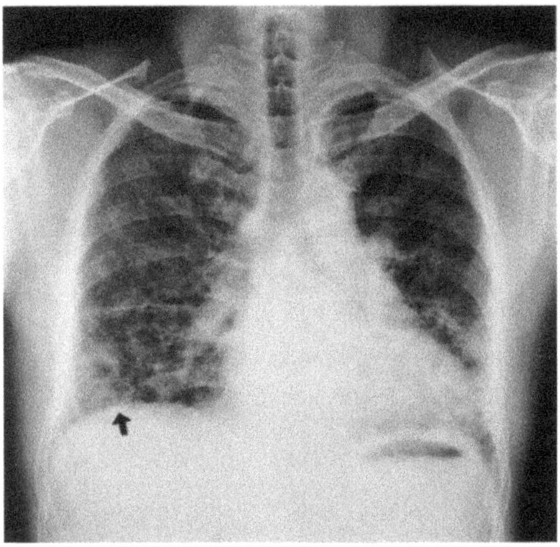

Fig. 9.38. A PA chest radiograph reveals dense distribution of irregular opacities in both middle and lower lung fields. Diffuse pleural thickening is noted in both lower zones, a finding typical of asbestos-related pleural disease. A calcified plaque is visible on the right hemi-diaphragm (*arrow*). The ILO classification is 2/2, s/s, ih, pc, pt

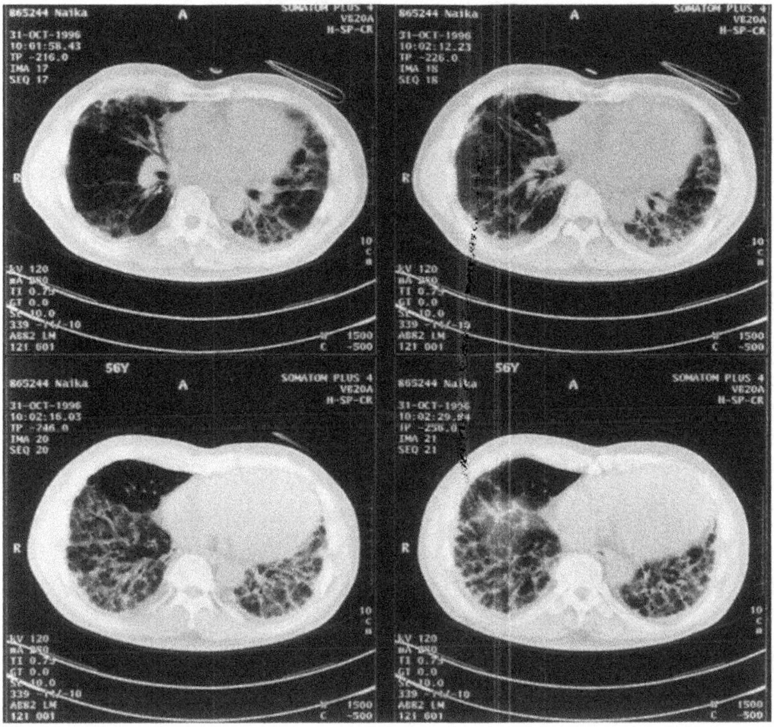

Fig. 9.39. CT images show diffuse interstitial fibrosis in both middle and lower lung zones

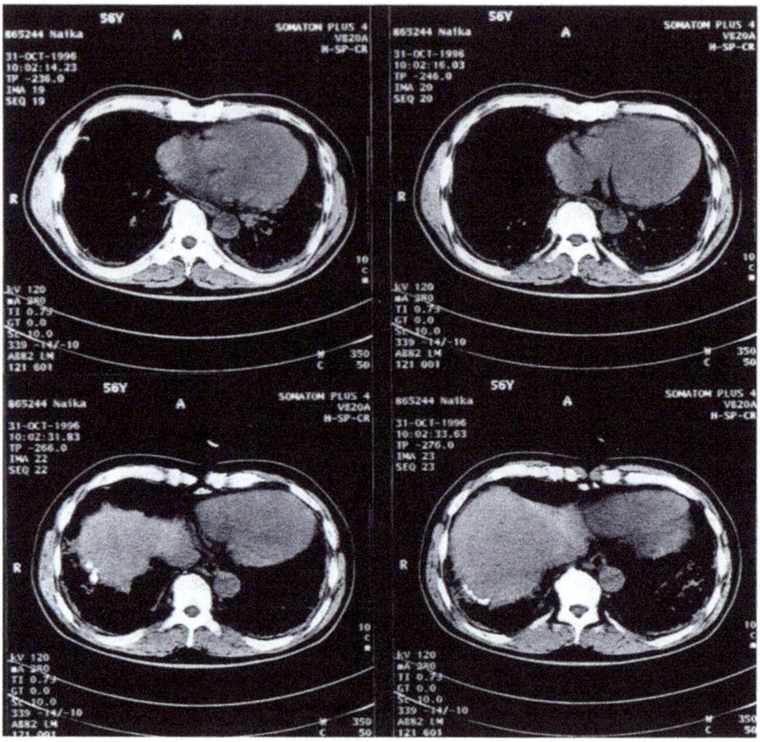

Fig. 9.40. CT images with mediastinal window setting demonstrate diffuse pleural thickening. Calcified plaque is noted on the right hemi-diaphragm

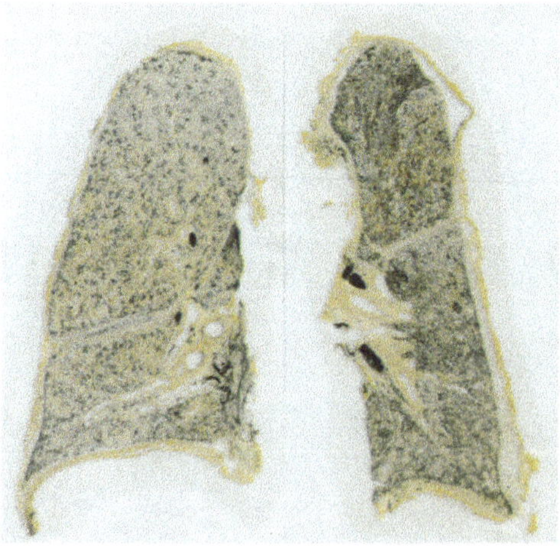

Fig. 9.41. Gough-Wentworth whole lung sections demonstrate diffuse interstitial fibrosis and markedly thickened pleurae

Histologic findings—

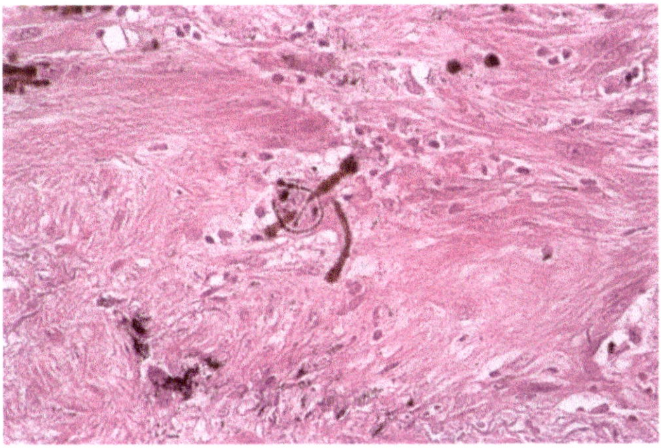

Fig. 9.42. Asbestos bodies deposited in the fibrotic tissue

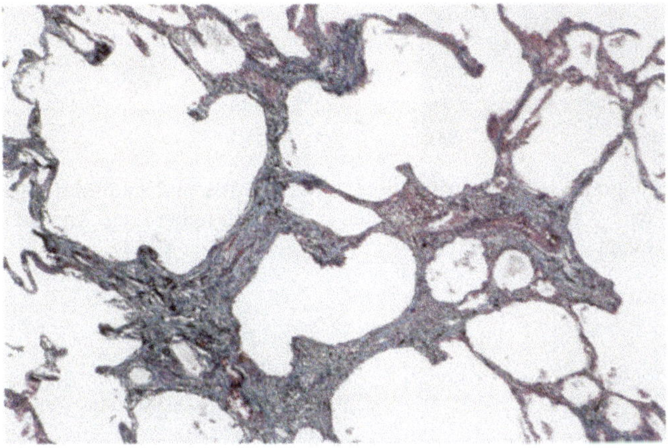

Fig. 9.43. Diffuse interstitial fibrosis with microscopic honeycombing

Case 8

A case of talco-asbestosis in a 68-year-old man who was engaged in crushing of diatomaceous earth and packing talcum powder in a talc factory for 13 years. Died of cor pulmonale.

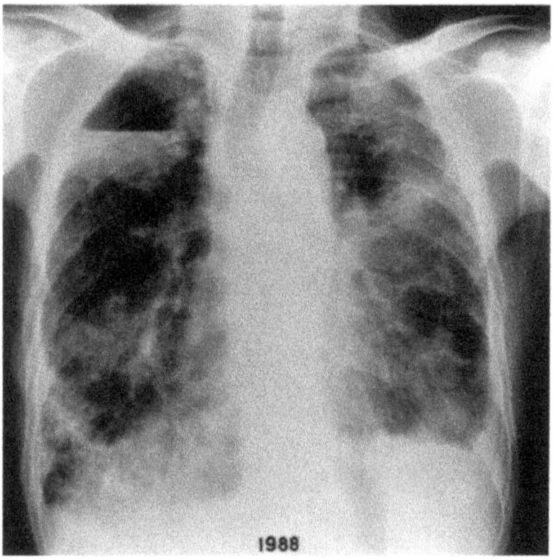

Fig. 9.44. A PA chest radiograph reveals diffuse interstitial fibrosis and multiple large opacities in both lungs. A cavity with fluid level is noted in the right upper lung. The ILO classification is C, 2/2, t/t, cv, pt

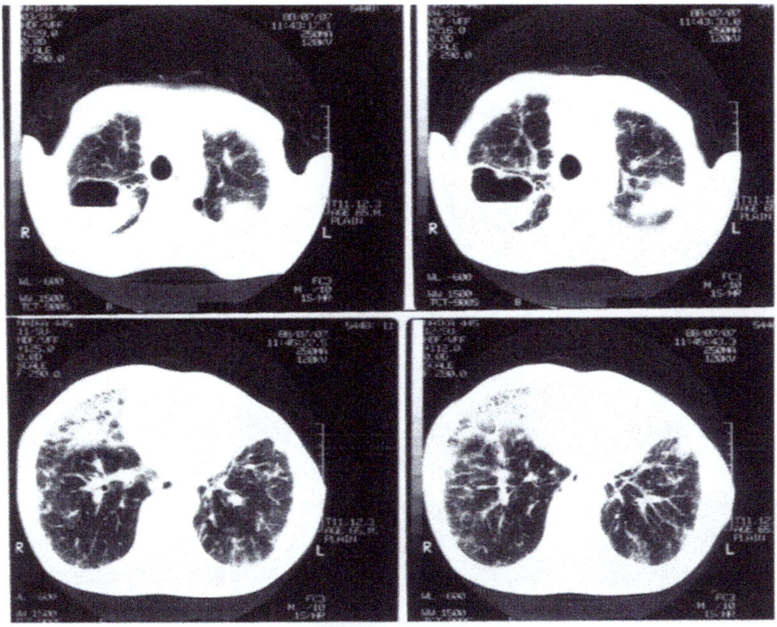

Fig. 9.45. CT images demonstrate a large cavity with fluid level in the right upper lung zone. In the lower zones, ground-glass and reticular opacities are noted bilaterally, suggesting diffuse interstitial fibrosis

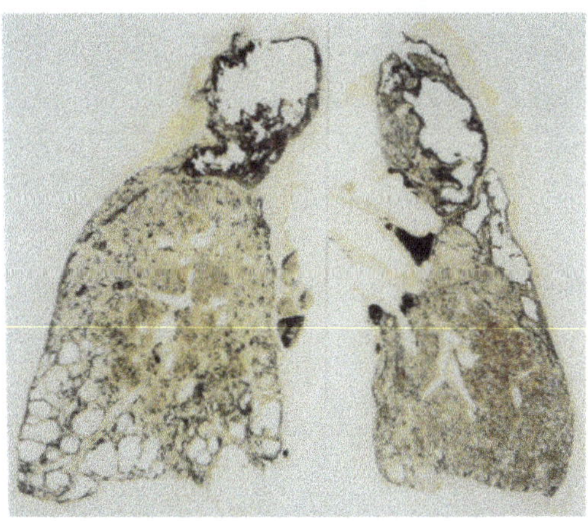

Fig. 9.46. Gough-Wentworth whole lung section demonstrates large pigmented cavitary masses in the upper lobes, diffuse interstitial fibrosis and marked honeycomb change involving the right lower lobe, sporadic pigmented fibrous nodules and diffuse pneumonic consolidations in the lower lobes

Histologic findings—

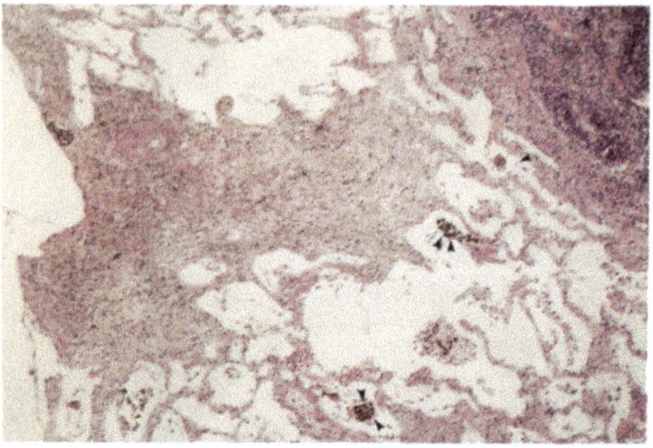

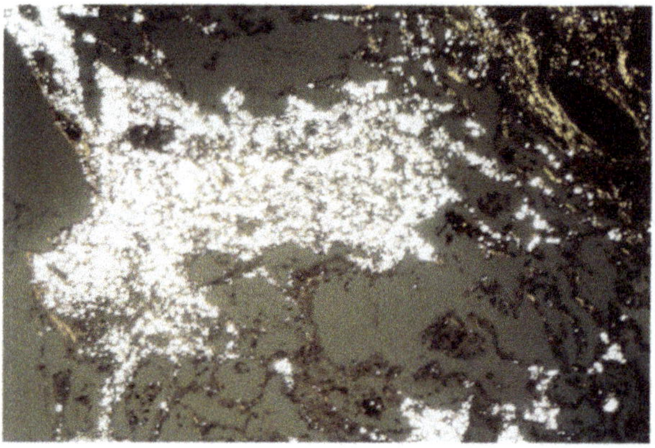

Fig. 9.47a, b. Talc granuloma is noted in the center of this image. Note the clusters of asbestos bodies in the alveoli (wedges) (a) and numerous birefringent talcum particles (b)

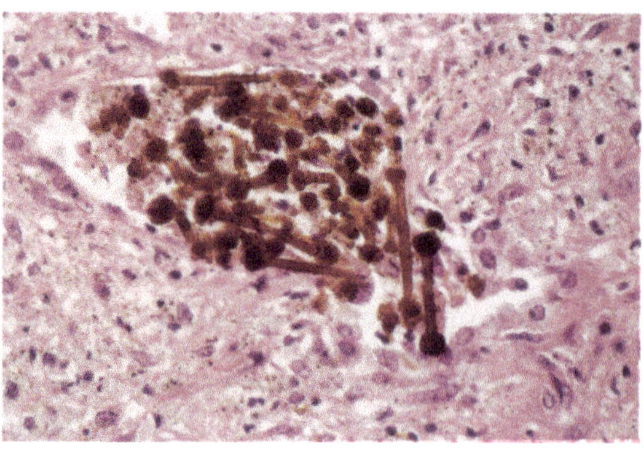

Fig. 9.48. A cluster of asbestos bodies surrounded by a fibrotic talc granuloma

References

1. Honma K, Abraham JL, Chiyotani K, De Vuist P, Dumortier P, Gibbs AR, Green FHY, Hosoda Y, Iwai K, Jones W, Kohyama N, Sstiguy G, Roggli VL, Shida H, Taguchi O, Vallyathan V. Nikko Criteria fro Mixed Dust Pneumoconiosis. Definition, Description and Guidelines for Pathologic Diagnosis and Clinical Correlation. J. Pulmo Pathol 2000; 1:1-13
2. Taguchi O, Saitoh Y, Saitoh K, Fuyuki T, Shida H, Mishina M, Chiyotani K, Honma K. Mixed dust fibrosis and tuberculosis in comparison with silicosis and macular pneumoconiosis. Am J Ind Med 2000; 37(3):260-4
3. Keizo C. Pneumoconiosis in 21st century in Japan. Jpn J Traum Occup Med 1999; 47:209-217
4. Shida H, Chiyotani K, Honma K, Hosoda Y, Nobechi T, Morikubo H, Wiot JF. Radiologic and pathologic characteristics of mixed dust pneumoconiosis. Radiographics 1996; 16(3):483-98

Subject Index

GPSR Compliance
The European Union's (EU) General Product Safety Regulation (GPSR) is a set of rules that requires consumer products to be safe and our obligations to ensure this.

If you have any concerns about our products, you can contact us on

ProductSafety@springernature.com

In case Publisher is established outside the EU, the EU authorized representative is:

Springer Nature Customer Service Center GmbH
Europaplatz 3
69115 Heidelberg, Germany

www.ingramcontent.com/pod-product-compliance
Ingram Content Group UK Ltd.
Pitfield, Milton Keynes, MK11 3LW, UK
UKHW020832270526
471509UK00003B/27
* 9 7 8 4 4 3 1 2 3 9 2 4 6 *